PENGUIN PASSNOTES

Nursing

David White, B. Sc. (Hons.), S.R.N., ̶, was educated at North London Polytechnic ̶ ̶ ̶ ̶ ̶ ̶ ̶ ̶ ̶ ̶ ̶ biology and chemistry. He trained as a general nurse at St George's Hospital, London, and after further training specialized in Intensive Care Nursing. He read for his Certificate in Education at Garnett College, London, and has subsequently taught the Basic Nursing Qualifications at the Wolfson School of Nursing of the Westminster Hospital.

Deliberate Self Harm · /DEPRESSION.
Renal
Drugs.

PENGUIN PASSNOTES

Nursing

DAVID WHITE, B.SC.(HONS.), S.R.N., R.M.N.,
CERT.ED.DIP.NURS.(LOND.)
ADVISORY EDITOR: STEPHEN COOTE, M.A., PH.D.

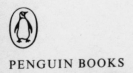

PENGUIN BOOKS

To Sally

Penguin Books Ltd, 27 Wrights Lane, London W8 5TZ (Publishing and Editorial)
and Harmondsworth, Middlesex, England (Distribution and Warehouse)
Viking Penguin Inc., 40 West 23rd Street, New York, New York 10010, USA
Penguin Books Australia Ltd, Ringwood, Victoria, Australia
Penguin Books Canada Ltd, 2801 John Street, Markham, Ontario, Canada L3R 1B4
Penguin Books (NZ) Ltd, 182–190 Wairau Road, Auckland 10, New Zealand

First published 1987
Reprinted 1988

Made and printed in Great Britain by
Richard Clay Ltd, Bungay, Suffolk
Filmset in Monophoto Times

Contents

Foreword

These Passnotes are written primarily for those students preparing for their final R.G.N. examination, although the notes may also be appropriate for the intermediate and modular tests and examinations which are set during the training programme.

It is not intended to be a textbook and should be used for revision purposes and not as a substitute for textbooks or tutorial and lecture notes.

The topics covered are all included in the current R.G.N. syllabus and they reflect the areas in which most students will gain experience and therefore the topics most commonly asked about in examination questions.

The first two chapters are concerned with methods of study and planning answers and the final chapter offers advice about what to do in the examination, and examination technique and preparation.

All the other chapters are on specific topics and most include an example of an essay answer and multiple choice questions in the subject area.

Acknowledgements

The publishers are grateful to the English and Welsh National Board for permission to reproduce examination questions. The multiple choice questions were validated by the Wolfson School of Nursing.

The Observation Chart reproduced on p. 119 was first published by G. Teasdale and B. Jennett in the issue of the *Lancet*, 2, 13 July 1974, pp. 81–4.

The author greatly acknowledges the help of Margaret P. Seymour, S.R.N., R.N.T., B.A.(Hons)Soc.Sci., Senior Tutor in Basic Education at the Royal Masonic and Roehampton Schools of Nursing; Michele B. Charles, S.R.N., R.S.C.N., R.C.N.T., R.N.T.Dip.Nurs.(Lond.), formerly Nurse Tutor, Wolfson School of Nursing; and Tess Ormrod, S.R.N., R.M.N., R.N.T., Senior Tutor in Post Basic Education, Hereford.

1. Introduction

1.1. The syllabus and examination (a) Aims of training 1.2. How to study 1.3. Use of this book 1.4. Answering questions (a) Reading the question; (b) Planning your answer; (c) Answering what is required; (d) General points 1.5. Sample question (answering technique)

1.1. The syllabus and examination

This book is written to cover the syllabus of training of the English and Welsh National Board for the qualification of Registered General Nurse (R.G.N.).

The content is also appropriate to the Scottish National Board syllabus but their examination structure is different and this should be noted by students using this book as a revision aid for Scottish Board examinations.

The current regulations of training for the English and Welsh Board R.G.N. examination are defined in terms of competencies.

Aims of training

The nurses' rules set out the objectives of the training programme for each level of registration.

The rules specify that courses leading to first-level registration shall provide opportunities to enable the student to accept responsibility for her personal professional development and to acquire the competencies required to:
(a) advise on the promotion of health and the prevention of illness;
(b) recognize situations that may be detrimental to the health and well-being of the individual;
(c) carry out those activities involved when conducting the comprehensive assessment of a person's nursing requirements;
(d) recognize the significance of the observations made and use these to develop an initial nursing assessment;

(e) devise a plan of nursing care based on the assessment with the co-operation of the patient to the extent that this is possible, taking into account the medical prescription;

(f) implement the planned programme of nursing care and where appropriate teach and co-ordinate other members of the caring team who may be responsible for implementing specific aspects of the nursing care;

(g) review the effectiveness of the nursing care provided and, where appropriate, initiate any action that may be required;

(h) work in a team with other nurses, and with medical and paramedical staff and social workers;

(i) undertake the management of the care of a group of patients over a period of time and organize the appropriate support services.

Examinations are currently being reviewed and an interim system is in operation. However, whether the examinations are set by the English and Welsh National Board or the schools of nursing on an individual basis, the content of the examination paper is likely to remain similar, although the format of the questions will vary with regard to style and length of time allowed for an answer.

You should ensure that you are familiar with the format of the final examination in use in the school of nursing in which you are training, e.g. are multiple choice items included? How long is allowed to answer the questions? What format do the questions take?

This book does not prepare you for internal practical assessments – whether of an individual or continuous type – but it may serve as a reference for considering the content of patient care plans that will be an important part of your assessment procedure.

1.2. How to study

Studying for examinations is very much an individual matter of choice. The following serve as guidelines and should be adapted to suit your needs.

As most students work a system of rotation duties including evening and night duty, it is best to identify the periods when you study best. Some students find that revising during their break on night duty is very useful while others cannot keep their eyes open at all. There are those who prefer to revise on their days off while others need this time to relax.

Whatever strategy you plan to follow, there are a number of points to remember.

(a) Planning your revision means sitting down and working out a schedule to cover the topics you need to revise for the examination. You may decide to follow the format of this book and revise the chapters on a regular basis.

(b) Having made a plan, it is important to try and keep to it. If you postpone topics because they are difficult, you will end up panicking as the examination date approaches as you have left too much to do.

(c) Decide how much time you are going to spend: for example, one hour five times per week. DO NOT commit yourself to working three to four hours per day every day as you will become too tired and your revision will be of much less benefit than if you revise regularly for short periods. DO NOT decide to cram it all into your last few days off before the examination as it is likely you will revise superficially.

(d) You may well wish to plan your revision in conjunction with submitting work to your tutor or in relation to your ward experiences and this will be useful reinforcement for the topics you are revising.

Remember, you have gained practical experience in nursing many patients, and relating this to the topic you are considering is necessary when revising.

(e) Choose an appropriate environment in which to revise. For many students, the only way to find a quiet place may be to go to the library of the school of nursing or a public library.

Do not try to revise while watching the television or chatting to your friends as you will not concentrate properly on your revision.

(f) Try to make sure you have eaten as otherwise you will be preoccupied with thinking about cooking supper rather than devoting your energies to your studies. If you need some coffee, make it before you start – do not sit down and then get up again after ten minutes to make it as this will interfere with your concentration.

(g) Revising with friends can be useful for some people but try to make sure you are studying properly and not just chatting.

(h) Make full use of tutors and clinical staff who can advise you if you are unsure of particular points.

(i) Try to enjoy your revision. When you achieve your targets reward yourself by, for example, going out for the rest of the evening.

Checklist of key points
1. Plan a revision programme and try to adhere to it.
2. Study regularly and not for too long at a time.
3. Carry out your study in a suitable environment.
4. Don't study to the exclusion of eating properly and relaxing.
5. Be disciplined in your approach.

1.3. Use of this book

The author has found that, at the time of writing, most students prefer to revise on 'system based' topics. The book has thus been presented in this way so as to allow the student to identify with this approach. Nursing is, however, now based on a problem-solving rather than a systems approach and this is considered under Nursing Models in Chapter 2.

When using this book, it is suggested that you use all of it rather than just refer to a specific chapter or topic if you wish to gain the most benefit from it. The chapters have been arranged to provide a logical sequence for study and are best considered in this way, e.g. Chapter 2 should be read before looking at Chapter 8.

Some limited cross-referencing takes place within the book.

The book should not be used to revise anatomy and physiology as this is outside the scope of the text. However, some inclusion is made, such as healing process in fractures, and there are some other very important diagrams.

There is also reference to a revision book which includes anatomy and physiology (*Penguin Masterstudies: Biology*) and students may find it useful to refer to this book.

Try to read the chapters before looking at the specimen questions or the multiple choice questions. The multiple choice answers are explained so as to help you understand the reasoning behind the correct answer. All questions have been pre-tested on students before inclusion.

When using this book it must be remembered that because all people are individuals, it is unlikely that their specific problems will be covered in only one chapter and thus you will need to transfer your learning of principles from a number of chapters when looking at previous examination questions. For example,

Q. Mr Clancy, aged 80 years, who has chronic bronchitis is admitted for a transurethral resection of prostate under a special anaesthetic.
(a) How can the nurse help him settle in the ward and provide specific psychological and physical preparation for surgery?   40%
(b) Describe the specific post-operative care Mr Clancy should receive to minimize the risk of complications during the first forty-eight hours.   60%
                    General Nursing Council for England and Wales, October 1982

An answer to this question requires information from Chapter 9 to cover his breathing problems, Chapter 7 about his preparation for surgery and Chapter 14 relating to his specific care following a transurethral resection.

1.4. Answering questions

In this section key points are identified in relation to the examination technique required for answering essay-style questions. These points are then illustrated by consideration of examination questions and the approach required to answer them.

The technique of problem solving is discussed in Chapter 2.

Reading the question

Always read through the question more than once before deciding to answer it.

Look carefully at the percentage weighting attached to each part.

Make sure you understand what the question is asking you about.

Do not attempt questions in which you are unsure of the meaning of words. For example, if the question asked is about 'iatrogenic' causes of illness in the elderly, do not write about 'ageing' in the elderly and hope this is correct as only part of your answer would cover iatrogenic (medically induced) causes of illness and you would be unlikely to gain enough marks to pass the question. Identify key words in the question, e.g. *sudden* dyspnoea; *extensive* burns; *elderly widow*; *acute* intestinal obstruction.

Planning your answer

This is very important especially if you are answering a 100 per cent essay question. You need to have an overall strategy to link the various points you are going to include in your answer. Very often by writing key words and/or facts on a piece of scrap paper or the answer paper, you can discover very quickly if you know enough about the topic to answer the question.

If the question asks for a problem-solving approach you can make a quick list of problems putting them in priority order and tick them off as you include them in your answer.

Ask yourself if specific points need to be included early in your answer and make your plan accordingly.

Once you have made an answer plan try to stick to it as if you branch away from it you may well end up including non-relevant material.

A good answer plan need only take a few minutes to prepare and can result in a far better answer than one which is written as the points are remembered.

Always put a line through rough working in your answer book so the examiner can clearly see that it is not part of your final answer.

Answering what is required

This is something which causes problems for many candidates. Do not be tempted to include irrelevant information as you will only waste time and gain no extra marks for it. If you have read the question properly and made an answer plan then it should be easier for you to see exactly what the examiner requires.

The wording of the question will give you a good indication of what is required and most questions are fairly explicit in this area. For example:

Q. Describe the nursing care during the first forty-eight hours following surgery.

The examiner only requires you to describe the nursing care during this period. You would not gain any more marks for discussing care after the first forty-eight hours.

Q. Describe the nursing observations while he is on bed rest.

You are being asked about the observations you make – what you look for and its significance. The type of treatment you carry out is not being asked for.

Q. Describe how Mr Johnson is orientated to the ward.

You need to consider the factors involved in orientating *him* and this would *not* include details of nursing admission/administration procedures unless relevant to *his* orientation.

Q. Identify complications which may develop and plan appropriate nursing measures.

This answer does not require you to give a general account of the relevant nursing care but requires you to identify the potential complications and then clearly show a plan of nursing action to deal with them.

Q. Explain how preoperative preparation reduces postoperative complication.

In this answer you must *explain* how your actions will achieve the end result, e.g. the teaching of deep breathing exercises prior to surgery. The examiner is not expecting you merely to give an account of pre- and postoperative care.

General points

(a) *Write legibly*. You must write your answer in such a way that the examiner is able to read it, otherwise it will not be possible for him to give you marks for your answer. An answer which is clearly written and with predominantly correct spelling is likely to impress much more than a poorly presented script with spelling mistakes which make the content ambiguous.

(b) *Comply with the instructions in the question*. For example, if the question uses words like list, plan, discuss, describe, explain principles, then you must do exactly that.

If you are asked to use a problem-solving approach then you must identify problems.

If the question asks you to explain how you would *teach* junior nurses, patients or relatives, remember to use appropriate language in your answer. The examiner is not only asking you what you know but also how you convey it to others.

(c) *Drawing diagrams*. If you are asked to illustrate your answer with a diagram, make sure it is clearly drawn and accurately labelled.

If you choose to use a diagram as part of your answer, then make sure it is relevant and really does illustrate the point you are trying to make. For instance, a diagram to illustrate balanced traction may well be better than a complicated written description.

(d) *Introductions and conclusions*. In 100 per cent essay answers, e.g. discussing the role of the nurse as a health educator, always start off with an introductory paragraph and finish with a concluding paragraph which summarizes your key points. This will give the examiner a good impression as he can see what you are intending to write about straight away and then be reminded of your key points at the end. It is important that your main content relates to the introduction and conclusion.

(e) *Using key words in the question*. If the question relates to a patient note his name, age, sex, marital status, and other relevant social information. The examiner will expect you to take this into account in your answer and it is a good idea to refer to it specifically at various stages in your answer to show you really are relating the answer to the question.

(f) *Don't waffle* – you will get no credit for long-winded paragraphs containing little or no information. It is not the number of words you write that is important but the content included in those words.

(g) *Be specific wherever possible.* For example, don't write: Observations were recorded. Write: The temperature, pulse and blood pressure were recorded two-hourly for twenty-four hours.

(h) *Avoid generalizations.* For example, 'General nursing care was given' – this type of statement could mean almost anything.

(i) *Avoid abbreviations* as they can be ambiguous or misunderstood. For example, don't write: Us and Es were done; write: blood was taken to measure urea and electrolyte levels.

Examples of specimen answers are given at the ends of most chapters and these include problem-solving approaches. The example that follows illustrates the relevant points identified in this chapter as well as including the appropriate content.

1.5. Specimen question (*answering technique*)

Q. *Mrs Wilson,* a 70-year-old widow, *lives alone in a rented flat. She is* overweight *and has a large gravitational ulcer on her leg. She has been* admitted in order to initiate *healing of the ulcer which has been enlarging recently.*

(a) *Based on the* principles *underlying the management of gravitational ulcers,* discuss *the care Mrs Wilson will require during her* first week *following admission.*   75%

(b) *What* advice *will Mrs Wilson require on discharge concerning the management of her ulcer at home?*   25%

Answering strategy

What are the key words? You may wish to write them down or underline them. (Gravitational = varicose.)

Plan
Care for the first week only
(a)

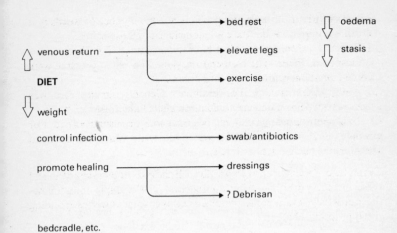

bedcradle, etc.

(*b*)
District nurse
Elevate legs
Bruising
Bandage/stockings
Diet/exercise

Specimen answer
(*a*) As the question asks you to discuss, based on principles, it is important that you do this and indicate the rationale for your nursing action. The answer is a discussion so it is probably better written in essay form and should be based on the following:
1. Improving venous return.
Action:
Bed rest initially (two or three days)
Leg elevated above the level of the heart
Elevate legs when sitting
Prevent crossing of legs
Prevent standing unless walking
Apply compression bandages, e.g. Ichthopaste, Viscopaste, Elastoplast, correctly when ulcer is clean/starting to heal. (Bandage from toes to knee.)
Rationale: The above all reduce circulatory stasis and venous congestion thereby relieving local oedema and improving cellular metabolism.
Action:
Encourage walking, ankle and calf exercises when leg is bandaged.

Rationale: Increase muscle pump action.

2. Reduce weight

Action:

Referral to dietitian

Dietary advice/education

Monitor weight regularly, e.g. weekly.

Rationale: To promote increased mobility and independence.

3. Good nutritional intake

Action:

Meals prepared in consultation with dietitian

Served attractively/small portions

Food she likes if possible

Good balanced diet.

Rationale: Adequate nutrients are necessary to allow healing and repair of damaged tissue. Balanced diet will also help reduce weight.

4. Control infection

Action:

Take wound swab and send to laboratory for microscope, culture and sensitivity.

Observe wound for evidence of infection, e.g. increased inflammation/discharge.

Administer prescribed antibiotics systematically and/or topically.

Use aseptic technique when carrying out dressings.

Rationale: The wound will not heal while it is infected.

5. Promote local healing

Action:

Keep the wound clean.

Cleanse and pack as is your hospital policy, e.g. use Debrisan, or Eusol and paraffin, or hydrogen peroxide and/or tulle gras.

Rationale: You would need to explain the rationale behind the method you suggest. For example, Debrisan beads are poured into the wound after cleansing with normal saline to a depth of 3 mm where they absorb the wound secretions by suction thereby removing bacteria and tissue debris and promoting healing.

6. Avoiding further damage

Action:

Use bedcradle.

Appropriate footwear.

Education of patient to avoid knocking legs.

Rationale: Further damage would cause healing to cease or be impaired.

(*b*) Advice on discharge should include:
ensuring patient understands arrangements for district nurse to visit
importance of walking and not standing, and of doing her exercises
wearing appropriate clothes/footwear
elevating her legs when sitting
avoiding knocking her leg
telling district nurse/general practitioner if she bruises it
trying to maintain nutritious diet
she must not interfere with or remove dressing/bandage
when healed, wear elasticated stockings
attending outpatients as required.

2. Care plans and problem solving

2.1. Introduction 2.2. Identifying problems 2.3. Setting aims/goals
2.4. Nursing action 2.5. Specimen R.G.N. question 2.6. Sample
question and answer

2.1. Introduction

Over the past few years the use of nursing models as a theoretical basis
for planning the care of patients has increased greatly. In some areas this
has been referred to as 'using the nursing process'.

Whether you have been taught or have gained practical experience on
the basis of one model, any number of different models or no model at
all makes no difference when you are answering problem-solving questions
as it is your ability to use a problem-solving approach that you are
required to demonstrate, not your knowledge of a particular theoretical
model of care.

You may wish to start your answer with, for example, 'This answer is
based on problems identified using the model of Roper's Activities of
Daily Living'. This obviously shows the examiner you have some
knowledge of nursing models, but remember to follow the model you
have specified if you choose this approach. It is unlikely that you would
be asked to answer a question using a named nursing model, e.g. *Using
Roy's model of nursing* ... However, if you are sitting an internally set
final examination it would be in your interest to have a good knowledge
of the model(s) used in your school of nursing and on the wards in which
you have been gaining experience, as you may be asked to relate your
answer specifically to an approach with which you would be expected to
be familiar.

All plans of care and descriptions of care must be related to the needs
or problems of the patient and the way in which the nurse can try to meet
these needs or resolve the problems. This is best achieved by identifying
clearly what the needs of the patient are and then planning the care
accordingly.

When answering questions this involves identifying the key words in the question carefully and then incorporating this information into your plan of care. You should also include the important points of care relating to the way in which you nurse patients with the particular condition.

The style in which you present the information is not important as long as you provide the information requested by the question.

If you are asked for a problem-solving approach then any of the below are acceptable examples of ways in which this can be done.

1. The problems are: (a); (b); (c); (d); (e); followed by a detailed account of the care required for each problem, or

2. Problem (a) followed by a detailed explanation of relevant care. This could then lead into problem (b) and so on throughout your answer, or

3.

Problem	Nursing goal/aim	Nursing action
1.	(a)	(i)
		(ii)
		(iii)
	(b)	(i)
		(ii)
2.	(a)	(i)
		(ii)

There are a number of ways in which you can divide the care up so as to ensure you include all aspects in your answer. The simplest is to separate it into three categories: physical, psychological, social, and to plan your answer under these headings. Alternatively, you can use one of the models of nursing with which you are familiar as a basis for your answer. For example, Activities of Daily Living,* as identified by Nancy Roper:

1. Maintaining a safe environment
2. Communicating
3. Breathing
4. Eating and drinking
5. Eliminating
6. Personal cleansing and dressing

*Roper, N., Logan, W. et al., *Elements of Nursing 1980* Churchill Livingstone, Medical Division, Longman Group 1984

7. Controlling body temperature
8. Mobilizing
9. Working and playing
10. Expressing sexuality
11. Sleeping
12. Dying.

or Patients' Needs,* as identified by Virginia Henderson.

1. Breathe normally.
2. Eat and drink adequately.
3. Eliminate body waste.
4. Move and maintain desirable postures.
5. Sleep and rest.
6. Select suitable clothes – dress and undress.
7. Maintain body temperature within normal range by adjusting clothing and modifying the environment.
8. Keep the body clean and well groomed and protect the integument.
9. Avoid dangers in the environment and avoid injuring others.
10. Communicate with others in expressing emotions, needs, fears or feelings.
11. Worship according to one's faith.
12. Work at something that provides a sense of accomplishment.
13. Play or participate in various forms of recreation.
14. Learn, discover or satisfy the curiosity that leads to normal development and health.

Whichever approach you use you need to ensure that you include all the relevant aspects of care the question has asked for. If you are using the above models remember that all patients do not always have problems with all of the points identified in the models and you need only include the relevant points for the specific patient whose care you are writing about.

If the question states that the patient is dyspnoeic and has a cough then you must include these problems when you are writing your care plan. A plan of care needs to have an ultimate objective. It should also have specific aims/goals which need to be achieved in order to obtain this objective.

For example, if Mr Jones has had a cerebrovascular accident leaving him with a right-sided weakness and you were planning his care from admission to discharge, the ultimate objective might be to help Mr Jones

*Published in *Basic Principles of Nursing Care*, © International Council of Nurses, PO Box 42, CH–1222, Geneva 20, Switzerland (1960)

to recover sufficiently in order to return to his home. The intermediate aims/goals would be very varied but would include assisting him with those needs which he could not at the present time satisfy without nursing help and intervention, as well as preventing complications which may occur as a result of his disability. For example, if we consider his difficulty with walking then the plan of care would include:

1. the initial care needed to prevent muscle wasting and spasticity;
2. the programme of gradual and progressive increases in exercises leading to mobility;
3. the multidisciplinary involvement in his rehabilitation programme;
4. the psychological support required.

Whichever format you use to present this information in your answer you will still be basing it upon a problem-solving cycle.

For example,

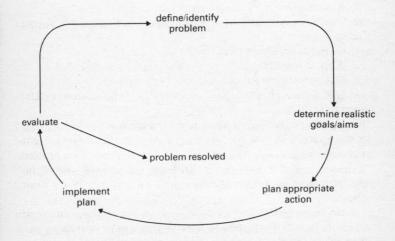

The fundamentals upon which individualized nursing care is based are:
1. Assessment – identifying problems
2. Planning – setting aims/goals
3. Implementation – nursing action
4. Evaluation of care given.

On the ward you obviously evaluate your care regularly as required and change your nursing action accordingly. In answer to an examination question you cannot evaluate theoretical care but you can indicate that you would do so. Thus, it is not sufficient to write

Problem	Aim	Nursing action
Pain in left leg	Relieve pain	Give analgesia as required

You need to be much more specific, for example: Give prescribed analgesia as required, e.g. Omnopon 10 mg intramuscularly and assess effect.

This shows the examiner that you understand the importance of evaluating care that you have planned.

2.2. Identifying problems

Make sure you know what type of problems you are being asked to identify. Are they
the patient's
the nurse's
physiological
psychological
social?

If the question asks you to *plan care using a problem-solving approach* then you can identify either the problems the patient has or the ones you will consider when giving your care.

If the question asks you to *identify Mr Smith's problems* then you must identify the problems *he* has and not yours.

In many cases the problems that you consider when planning care are exactly the same as those the patient complains of but not always. For example, both the nurse and the patient should always identify difficulty in breathing and inability to maintain an adequate airway as a major problem. But the patient would not identify the maintenance of his fluid balance status as a major problem for him unless he experienced the effects of the imbalance, e.g. thirst. The nurse however must consider this as an important aspect of care irrespective of whether imbalance occurs or not.

One method of clearing up the difficulty of how to include this information in an answer specifically related to patient problems is to identify the problems in two categories:

1. Actual – those present at the time of assessment
2. Potential – those which may develop if certain nursing action is not taken.

Using the example above, the patient has *potential* problems of (a) circulatory overload, and (b) dehydration. This then allows you to include the relevant nursing action in your answer while still presenting it in the way asked for in the question.

2.3. Setting aims/goals

Once you have identified the problems you can now set the nursing care goals. These must relate to the problems you have identified and can be very straightforward:

Problem	Goal
Constipation	Relieve constipation

or may consist of a number of stages:

Problem	Goal
Hypothermia	(a) Restore normal body temperature
	(b) Maintain normal body temperature
	(c) Patient maintains own body temperature herself.

In example 2 above, the question might have asked for detailed care in relation to an elderly lady suffering from exposure and it would be important for you to show you understood the different nursing actions to take at the various stages of her recovery.

2.4. Nursing action

This is what you would actually do and can be presented in paragraph or plan form when using a problem-solving approach.

It is important to show the examiner that you understand why you are carrying out the particular actions and you may be asked specifically in some questions to include a rationale for your action. This can be included with the nursing action or recorded in a separate column.

Remember to ensure that your proposed action is appropriate to the problem you have identified.

Problem	Aim	Nursing action	Rationale
Dyspnoea	Relieve dyspnoea	1. Sit patient upright supported by pillows	Reduces pressure from abdominal organs and allows easier expansion of the lungs
		2. Give humidified O_2 and bronchodilators as prescribed	Humidification loosens secretions and prevents air passages drying. Bronchodilators relieve bronchospasm and thus allow increased oxygenation

or

Problem	Aim	Nursing action	Rationale
Pyrexia	Reduce temperature to within normal limits	1. Remove bedclothes other than a cotton sheet	To promote heat loss by radiation and convection
		2. Dress in loose cotton pyjamas/nightdress	
		3. Ensure room is cool with good ventilation	
		4. Use tepid sponging or a cold air fan as prescribed	
		5. Measure and record body temperature, e.g. two-hourly	To assess effect of actions 1–4

The nursing action taken must obviously relate to the specific patient being asked about in the question and the way in which this is done is best considered by looking at the specimen care plan answers to questions at the ends of many of the chapters.

A general problem-solving answer is included here to illustrate the principles and to show how specific problems can be considered in detail when writing answers and planning care.

2.5. Specimen R.G.N. question

Q. Mr John Foot, aged 36 years, sustained a head injury when he fell from a ladder while cleaning windows. He is now in the trauma ward and is unconscious.

Identify Mr Foot's likely problems while he is unconscious and describe the observations the nurse should make, including their significance.

100%

Final R.G.N. paper, English and Welsh National Board, November 1984

2.6. Sample question and answer

Q. Mrs Ethel Johnson is a 47-year-old lady who is admitted to your ward suffering from acute liver failure. She has lost weight and feels lethargic. She has had an episode of haematemesis and malaena and is complaining of abdominal discomfort.

Using a problem-solving approach plan the nursing care in detail with particular reference to her gastrointestinal problems.   100%

Plan
Problems identified in question:
weight loss (due to anorexia/poor diet)
lethargy
haematemesis
malaena
abdominal discomfort.
Other gastrointestinal problems associated with acute liver failure and relevant to Mrs Johnson are:
nausea and vomiting
diarrhoea.

Problem	Aim	Nursing action
Weight loss	1. Encourage appetite. 2. Prevent further weight loss. 3. Maintain appropriate weight.	(a) Present food attractively and in small portions at frequent intervals. (b) Encourage patient to eat food she prefers. (c) Supplement food with high-calorie drinks. (d) Give prescribed vitamin supplements, e.g. Parentrovite. (e) Monitor weight regularly to assess effect of (a)–(e), e.g. twice weekly.
Lethargy	Help patient to make best use of her reduced energy	(a) Encourage high-calorie/build-up foods to increase her energy. (b) Do not overtire patient by allowing unnecessary physical expenditure of her energy. (c) Ensure her locker and bed table are within easy reach. (d) Help her to use a bedpan and to wash.
Haematemesis	Minimize the effects of episodes of haematemesis by: 1. Early detection	(a) Observe for signs indicative of gastrointestinal bleeding. (b) Monitor vital signs, e.g. temperature, pulse, respiration, blood pressure, central venous pressure, frequently, depending upon her condition, e.g. half-hourly or hourly. (c) Record volume of blood vomited and whether it was fresh blood or partially digested.

Problem	Aim	Nursing action
	2. Promoting comfort	(a) Try to provide as quiet an environment for the patient as possible.
		(b) Encourage rest.
		(c) Give frequent mouthwashes, e.g. hourly and after bleeding.
		(d) Position patient as comfortably as her cardiovascular status permits.
		(e) Ensure nightdress and bed linen are changed following haematemesis if dirty.
	3. Carrying out prescribed medical treatment and associated nursing care	(a) Carry out appropriate observations in relation to administration of a blood transfusion with regard to the safety and prevention of complications. (See chapter 16 for further details.)
		(b) Carry out care appropriate to the presence of a nasogastric tube or a Sengstaken tube.
		(c) Administer drugs, e.g. vitamin K to assist with blood clotting.
		(d) Administer drugs, e.g. lactulose, and magnesium sulphate designed to reduce the protein load from digestion of blood by promoting diarrhoea.
		(e) Administer drugs, e.g. Neomycin to kill bacteria in the bowel (protein source).

Problem	Aim	Nursing action
Malaena	Minimize the effects of malaena by:	
	1. Early detection	(a) Observe stools for colour and presence of malaena.
		(b) Record volume and time when stool passed.
		(c) Monitor changes in vital signs as in haematemesis, 1.
	2. Promoting comfort	(a) Ensure nightdress and bed linen are changed following malaena if dirty.
		(b) Use protective measures, e.g. Incopads.
		(c) Wash patient appropriately following malaena.
		(d) Apply Vaseline to anus to help prevent soreness.
		(e) Position patient as comfortably as cardiovascular status permits.
Abdominal discomfort	Relieve discomfort	(a) Change position of patient as often as required to increase her comfort.
		(b) Ensure she rests on her bed so as to reduce workload on the liver.
		(c) Administer antispasmodic drugs and possibly mild analgesia as prescribed and assess effect.
		(d) Encourage patient to eat slowly.

Problem	Aim	Nursing action
Nausea and vomiting	Relieve nausea and vomiting	(a) Administer prescribed antiemetics and assess effect. (b) Administer prescribed parenteral nutrition as an alternative to oral feeding if this is not possible. (c) Ensure regular mouth care is carried out prior to meals and following episodes of vomiting. (d) Ensure vomit bowl and tissues are easily available for patient's use.
Diarrhoea	Relieve diarrhoea (unless deliberately induced, see haematemesis, 3d)	(a) Administer prescribed medication, e.g. Lomotil and assess effect. (b) Ensure adequate fluid intake to prevent dehydration due to diarrhoea.

When answering this question it would be appropriate to start with an introductory paragraph explaining your approach. For example, 'A care plan based on the following problems ...', or 'Treatment and nursing action for haematemesis and malaena will vary depending on severity and frequency of episodes ...'

3. Care of children

3.1. Introduction

This chapter is intended to give guidelines concerning the many special
factors which must be taken into account when planning care for children.
A child has unique needs, dependent upon matters such as his age,
sex, stage of development, family and community background, past
experiences and upbringing. In relation to illness, the acuteness or chronicity of his condition must also be considered. The way in which these
needs are met during a period of hospitalization can have a long-lasting
effect upon the child, and so the importance of this subject cannot be
overstated.

It is not the intention of this chapter to give details of various paediatric
illnesses, although mention may be found of some childhood conditions
in chapters dealing with specific disorders, e.g. childhood fractures are
discussed in Chapter 13. It is not expected that R.G.N. students will have
a detailed knowledge of paediatric medicine; where an examination
question relating to children mentions a specific illness, it will generally
be a common one found on the average paediatric ward. It may be a
condition which also affects adults; however, it is quite insufficient when
writing about a child simply to give a 'scaled-down' version of the care

you would give the adult. In your answer, you will be expected to demonstrate in practical terms that you have considered the special needs of the child. Pointers are given on ways in which common aspects of nursing care can be adapted or altered to suit the needs of children of various ages.

The chapter concludes with some sample questions and answers.

3.2. Normal child growth and development; detection of abnormalities

You should have a fairly good knowledge of the normal sequence of child growth and development, and be aware of the 'milestones' of development with the usual ages at which these are reached. It is not expected that you will have the very detailed knowledge of an R.S.C.N. student, and more help can be obtained by studying the sections and charts on child development found in chapters on paediatric nursing in general textbooks, or in books on paediatric nursing written for general nurses, e.g. B. F. Weller and S. Barlow, *Paediatric Nursing* (Nurses' Aids Series), 6th ed., Baillière Tindall, 1983.

To aid revision, a summary of normal growth and development is given below, and you will see that there are many categories of development which have to be considered

Early childhood (0–5 years)

(See chart on pp. 36–8)

Middle childhood (6–9 years)

Develops co-ordination of fine muscles, becoming skilful in manual activities, and achieves grace and balance even in active sports. The family atmosphere has a great impact on the child's emotional development and he needs help in adjusting to new experiences and demands. He usually has a wide circle of friends at school. He is capable of making simple generalizations and elementary verbal reasoning, and is able to form some abstract concepts.

Late childhood (9–12 years)

The child begins to take on a more adult appearance: in females the development of secondary sexual characteristics and the growth spurt

Age	Physical growth and development	Posture and movement	Vision and manipulation	Hearing and speech	Social development
Birth – 1 month	Weight: 3.4 kg Length: 50 cm Head circumference: 33 cm at birth	Has primitive reflexes – sucking, grasping, responds to sudden sounds. By 1 month, raises head slightly from prone	By 1 month, follows object to midline		By 1 month regards face of parent or other handler
3 months	Weight: 5 kg	Lifts up head and chest when prone. Makes crawling movements	Follows dangling toy from side to side	Listens to interesting sounds. Squeals with pleasure	Responds to mother's smile. Smiles with pleasure
6 months	Weight: 7.5 kg First teeth erupt	Rolls from back to front. Sits with support	Turns head to increase visual field. Reaches out and grasps toy; puts to mouth	Babbles and makes tuneful sounds	Alert; friendly with strangers. Loves repetitive games, e.g. peek-a-boo
9 months	Weight: 9.5 kg Four upper incisors erupt	Wriggles or crawls prone. Sits unsupported for ten minutes	Looks for dropped toys. Has scissor grasp and transfers to other hand	Imitates sounds, says 'dada/mama' inappropriately	Distinguishes strangers with apprehension. Chews solids

Age	Physical growth and development	Posture and movement	Vision and manipulation	Hearing and speech	Social development
1 year	Weight: 10.5 kg Length: 73 cm Head circumference: 46 cm Six teeth present	Crawls on all fours; walks with one hand held. Stands alone for a few seconds	Drops toys deliberately and watches where they fall. Has pincer grasp	Uses two words with meaning. Obeys simple commands	Imitates actions; co-operates with dressing. May be shy
1½ years	Anterior fontanelle closed. Has fourteen teeth	Walks alone, throws ball from standing without falling	Turns pages of book; builds a three-block tower. Begins to use a spoon	Uses about ten words with meaning. Points to named body parts	Interested in strangers; wants to explore everything. Plays alone near others
2 years	Weight: 11–12 kg Height: 86 cm Head circumference: 48 cm Has sixteen to twenty teeth. Has bladder control	Runs. Walks up and down steps two feet to a step without help	Builds a tower of six cubes. Turns pages singly. Can open doors	Uses fifty words, says sentences of two or three words. Names objects in pictures	Helps actively to dress or undress. Indicates toilet needs. Parallel play, watches others play
3 years	By 2½ years has full set of primary teeth	Pedals tricycle. Uses alternate feet on stairs. Jumps and balances on one foot	Feeds himself well. Dries hands if reminded. Strings large beads	Uses plurals, and past tense. Tells short stories about experiences. Knows own sex	Will share toys, play well with others and take turns. Often has imaginary friend

Age	Physical growth and development	Posture and movement	Vision and manipulation	Hearing and speech	Social development
4–5 years	By 5 years: Height: 108 cm Weight: 18 kg	Hops and skips. Good motor control – climbs and jumps well	Matches simple shapes, builds three steps from six cubes after demonstration. Copies a O and X; later copies □ Prints first name	Talks a lot. Has fluent speech with few infantile substitutions. Knows colours. Counts to ten. Recites rhymes and songs	Buttons and unbuttons clothes. By 5 years, ties shoelaces. Goes to toilet alone. Prefers group play
6 years	Growth rate slow and steady	Balance improves	Draws a man, copies a ◇. Draws large letters or figures	Spells and reads simple words. Can repeat five digits	Enjoys constructive play, e.g. brick-building, plasticine modelling

occurs at 10 to 12 years; in males it occurs a little later at 12 to 14 years. The child works hard to perfect physical skills, and co-operates well with companions – he often has several close 'chums'. He has various hobbies and makes collections of objects. The child enjoys reasoning, and though thinking is still mostly in concrete terms, by the end of the period he begins conceptual thinking.

Early adolescence (13–15 years)

During the growth spurt the skeletal system grows faster than the supporting muscles and the large muscles develop more quickly than the small ones, so the teenager often appears uncoordinated and clumsy with poor posture. The peer group or 'gang' becomes more important than the family, and usually the gang is single-sex at this age. Behaviour tends to conform to the standards of the peer group, and interests usually include sports, music, T.V. and 'going out with the gang'. The teenager begins to use foresight and judgement, and to learn from experience. He is capable of highly imaginative thinking and has a wide range of knowledge.

Late adolescence (16–18 years)

Physical growth is completed and the teenager regains co-ordination and strength. Peer groups are still important, but attention turns towards the opposite sex and dating usually starts with groups of couples progressing to single couples. Intellectual development is nearing completion, and the adolescent develops goals, ideals and sentiments. He is capable of making sensible adaptations to present situations and planning for the future.

A knowledge of these normal patterns of growth and development helps the nurse to have reasonable expectations of children, plan suitable activities and play within the limits and capabilities of the child, and also be alert to identify abnormalities, handicap and regression. However, it should be remembered that there is a considerable range of 'normal' patterns, e.g. babies may start walking at any time between 9 and 14 months. There may also be differences depending on race, culture and social class – Oriental children may be rather smaller than their Caucasian counterparts, and children of intellectual parents who have spent considerable time teaching them may learn to read much earlier than those from homes with few books and busy parents. Therefore, a variety of other factors have to be taken into account when assessing what is 'normal' for the individual child.

3.3 The needs of the child and the family

While a child has unique and special needs, he is part of a family unit, and so his needs will be intricately tied up with the needs and lifestyle of the whole family. Therefore, when planning to meet the needs of a child the rest of the family must be considered and as closely involved as possible. The goal in paediatric nursing is family-centred care. In practical terms this often means the mother playing the most important role, but the rest of the family must not be forgotten.

The child has biological needs common to all human beings – warmth, comfort, food, clothing, shelter and rest – but in order to thrive, the child also has the vital needs of love, security, affection and approval. The relative strengths of these needs and the exact manner in which they can be fulfilled will, of course, depend upon the child's age, stage of development and the particular circumstances, as can be inferred from the table. For example, a newborn baby needs the security of having a capable and dependable care-giver meet his biological needs. A 6- to 9-month-old baby, aware of his mother and apprehensive of strangers, particularly needs maternal love and affection. A toddler needs an environment of consistent family love and discipline to enable him to start to explore his surroundings. School-age children need help and understanding to adjust to new situations, with family and friends in the background. Teenagers need the security of the approval and company of their peer group, together with understanding of their emotional lability and opportunities for independence.

Children of all ages need opportunities for play and activities to help them practise and consolidate existing skills, while reaching out to develop new skills in all the categories of motor, language and social development. Thus, to meet the needs for play appropriately, the nurse must know the present level of development and the next stages in development to be attained.

3.4. The child in the community; recognition of the child 'at risk'

A child and his family are part of a community and so in planning effective care for a child, details of his community background must be found out and taken into consideration. Community environment includes such things as geographical location, the type and layout of housing, the atmosphere, and cultural and racial influences. Side by side in a paediatric ward you may encounter a child from a large Asian family living in one-room, bed-and-breakfast council accommodation in the heart of a big city, and the only child of fairly wealthy parents living in a large converted farmhouse in the countryside. While both children may be suffering from the same condition, such as a fractured tibia and fibula, their problems will obviously be rather different. The Asian child's parents may find it difficult to visit frequently because of financial hardship and caring for the rest of the family, and he may feel very isolated in a strange place, especially if his English is rather poor. His leg may fail to heal well because of a diet lacking in vitamin D, and it might be difficult to provide him with suitable food to meet his cultural and dietary requirements. His parents will have many problems caring for him in one room in bed-and-breakfast accommodation if he is discharged in a wheelchair. On the other hand, the child of wealthy parents may find it very strange to have to sleep in a ward full of other children, although his mother can stay with him, and he may miss the countryside and resent the enforced inactivity.

There are quite a number of facilities available in the community for the care of children, and you should be aware of these. If an examination question asks you to discuss care of a child after he returns home, or preparation for discharge, you may need to mention appropriate community provisions. Ensure that you know a little about the roles of each of the following:

child health clinics
health visitors
general practitioners
day nurseries
residential nurseries
nursery schools
play groups
crèches
school health service
child guidance clinics
special schools for mentally and physically handicapped children
social worker.

A considerable number of charities exist to look after the interests of children. Many of these are concerned with families and children with special needs, e.g. Association for Spina Bifida and Hydrocephalus (A.S.B.A.H.), but others are concerned with the welfare of children in general. Examples of these are:

National Children's Bureau
National Association for Maternal and Child Welfare

National Society for the Prevention of Cruelty to Children (N.S.P.C.C.)
National Association for the Welfare of Children in Hospital
(N.A.W.C.H.)
Mention can be made of the ways in which these can offer support and
help where appropriate.

In addition, a range of benefits is available under certain circumstances
to help families with the care of children. Some of these benefits are
specifically for the care of sick or handicapped children. They include:
Supplementary Benefit
Family Income Supplement
free milk and vitamins
free school meals
education benefits
attendance allowance
house adaptation and equipment
assistance with transport costs, or Mobility Allowance.
Nurses should be aware of the range of benefits available so that they can
liaise with social workers in ensuring that the family receives all the
support to which it is entitled.

It is very important that all nurses should be alert to the signs which
indicate that a child is 'at risk' from some form of non-accidental injury,
abuse or deprivation. The nurse is often in the best position to spot these,
whether in the community, casualty department or the paediatric ward,
and prompt reporting of worrying signs can help to prevent tragedies.
Evidence of a knowledge of these is sometimes looked for in examination
answers and multiple choice questions.

The various categories of child abuse, together with alerting signs, are
summarized below:
1. *Physical injury*:
(a) History doesn't adequately account for injury
(b) Delay in seeking help
(c) Repeated visits to doctor or hospital for injuries
(d) New and old lesions present, e.g. bruises, fractures
(e) Typical injuries – bite marks, belt marks, cigarette burns, finger-tip
bruising, two black eyes
(f) Sometimes accompanying evidence of neglect.
(g) Characteristic cowed, watchful expression on child's face, described
as 'frozen awareness'.
2. *Physical neglect*:
Persistent or severe signs of neglect, including exposure to dangers of

different kinds such as cold and starvation; failure to provide medical care.

3. *Failure to thrive*:

Severe non-organic failure to thrive, including emotional deprivation affecting behaviour and emotional development. Children may be left locked in rooms, constantly terrorized or berated, or totally rejected.

4. *Sexual abuse*:

From a close relative or care-giver.

Other children in a household where one child has been abused can also be considered 'at risk'.

Predisposing factors for child abuse have been identified as:

1. Poverty and poor housing
2. Overcrowding and large families
3. Unemployment
4. Immature parents, from broken homes themselves
5. Parents may also have been abused as children
6. Marital problems
7. Unwanted, unplanned child
8. Child who is a poor feeder and cries a lot
9. Handicapped child
10. Young children, under 2, most at risk
11. Lack of bonding with child owing to separation after birth, e.g. because of low birth-weight, respiratory problems
12. Mental illness in parents in 10 per cent of cases.

Usually a combination of several of these factors is present in the background of children who are abused, and a knowledge of these factors is helpful in alerting a nurse to the possibility of abuse if the child appears to have an unusual injury.

3.5 Effects of illness and handicap on children

The effects of an illness or handicapping condition on a child and his family vary according to the nature of the condition, and the resources of the family and individual to cope with it. These factors must also be borne in mind when assessing the needs of the sick child and planning care.

An *acute illness* is one which arises abruptly in a previously healthy child. Children can become ill very quickly (and recover just as quickly!). Apart from specific symptoms, behavioural signs that a child is acutely ill include:

regression to more childish behaviour
passive acceptance of treatment
cannot be distracted if in severe pain
unresponsive to people and objects around him.

Different age-groups manifest some specific behaviours indicating acute illness.

1. *Babies*:
(a) Different cry and posture
(b) Reluctance to feed
(c) Anxious attachment to mother in older baby over 6 months.

2. *Toddlers*:
(a) Actions indicating discomfort, e.g. excessive thumb-sucking
(b) Lack of normal inquisitiveness
(c) No normal distress at mother's departure.

3. *Pre-schoolers*:
(a) Complain of generalized pain
(b) Little interest in play
(c) Regression to earlier habits, e.g. bed-wetting.

4. *School-age children*:
(a) Communication of pain and other symptoms
(b) Accept help with care normally carried out for themselves.

5. *Adolescents*:
(a) Need the same degree of comfort and attention as younger children
(b) May react aggressively or become withdrawn.

The family also has to adjust and possibly change plans in view of a child's sudden illness. Where the illness is very serious or requires emergency surgery, there is the added worry about the outcome. There is little or no time to prepare the child for hospitalization and treatment, and so the child needs extra explanations and reassurance, and whenever possible the presence of a parent staying in the hospital with him. Other siblings may miss the ill child, and be frightened that they will develop the same illness.

A *chronic disease* is an illness which continues to damage the body over a long period of time and in children is usually associated with an underlying abnormality, e.g. cystic fibrosis. Chronic childhood disease affects all members of the family and may require a considerable change in lifestyle, e.g. to accommodate the child's treatment or frequent hospital visits. The parents may become rather over-protective with the child, perhaps fearing to punish him in case it exacerbates his condition. The child may discover how to manipulate this to his own advantage, and consequently become spoilt and naughty. The parents, especially the mother, may devote so much time to the chronically ill child that other siblings become neglected and jealous and marital difficulties can arise between the parents. Because of adaptations in their lifestyle and problems with participation in normal community events, the family and child may become socially isolated. Schooling may be a problem, although there is increasing emphasis on trying to integrate children with special needs into normal schools. In a few cases, a child with a chronic disease may be rejected by his parents.

As the chronicity of the disease and the limitations which it will place on his lifestyle become apparent to the older child, he may try to deny it and refuse treatment, or react with aggression and depression. The nurse must understand the reason for these reactions and help the child to work through them towards acceptance of his condition.

A *handicap* is a disability which, for a substantial period or permanently, retards, distorts, or otherwise affects normal growth, development or adjustment to life. Some handicaps are congenital – present at birth – e.g. spina bifida, while others are acquired later on, e.g. due to accidents. Especially where the handicapping condition is congenital, the parents and family have to 'mourn' for the loss of the expected normal child before they can accept the handicapped one. Handicaps are often visually apparent and of a more severe nature than chronic illness, and thus while many of the problems are common to both categories, there is likely to be greater hardship in cases of handicap. Emotional stress may be pronounced; commonly parents worry about how they will cope as they get older, and what will happen to their child when they die. Financial hardship is also more likely, as it is costly to provide care for a handicapped child at home. As the child gets older and develops his own self-image, he may be acutely embarrassed by his handicap and isolate himself, fearing the reactions of the public. The nurse needs to remember that handicapped children have all the normal needs of other children, although they also have some special needs, and the way in which some of the physical needs are met may have to be adapted to suit the individual child. Therefore, when answering a question which details a medical condition, it is necessary to determine into which category the condition falls, and then to remember the likely effect it will have on the child and the family, and plan care accordingly.

3.6. Admission of a child to hospital; ways of minimizing the adverse effects of hospitalization

A period of hospitalization can have a very marked effect on a child's development, and since first impressions count for a good deal the way in which the child and his parents are admitted to hospital is one crucial factor in determining how the child will adjust to his hospital stay. As surveys have shown that

1. a quarter of all children in this country will go into hospital before the age of 5; and

2. almost half of the nation's children will have been patients by the age of 7,

this subject is obviously an important one, and is frequently asked about in examination questions on the care of children. (For examples, see the sample questions at the end of this chapter.)

The ability of a child to adapt to hospital depends on:

1. his age and emotional maturity
2. security in his home environment
3. previous traumatic experiences
4. attitude of his parents
5. preparation for coming into hospital
6. nature of his illness
7. length of hospital stay
8. quality of care in hospital from the time of admission onwards.

While nurses cannot influence some of the above factors, such as 1, 2, 3 and 6, they must find out about them and bear them in mind. Factors 4 and 5 can be influenced partially by nurses, both by those whom parents and children may encounter in the community, and those whom they meet in the outpatients department and wards. Good nursing care may help to limit 7, and certainly nurses play a major role in influencing 8.

Ideally, the child should be well prepared in advance for coming into hospital. *General preparation* about hospitals can begin very early, especially as many children may be admitted in an emergency without time for specific preparation. This can take the form of

1. general conversations about hospitals, doctors, nurses, ambulance sirens, etc;

2. hospital stories, e.g. Althea (1974) *Going to the hospital*, Dinosaur Publications;

3. playing doctors and nurses with dolls, uniform for dressing up, miniature 'medical kits';

4. avoiding using hospital as a punishment threat.

Specific preparation for a known hospital admission may include:
1. a visit to the hospital; tour of the ward and meeting staff if possible;
2. reading the hospital booklet, colouring in pictures;
3. parental information from hospital leaflets, N.A.W.C.H. publications, etc;
4. if the child has never slept away from home before, perhaps spending one or two nights with grandparents, friendly neighbour; and
5. encouraging the child to help pack a case to take into hospital, choosing favourite toys to take with him and putting name labels on them. A small practical present can be bought as a present to take into hospital, e.g. new pyjamas. The child can organize some things ready for his return, so that he knows he will be coming back.

Preparations for the child's *admission in the ward* include :
1. selecting the most appropriate area of the ward, depending on age, sex and condition, and preparing the cot/bed area, perhaps putting a suitable toy on the bed
2. selecting the nurse who will play a major role in caring for the child – he/she should be the one to greet and admit the child;
3. finding out details about the child in advance, so he and his parents can be greeted by name.

The admission begins when the child and his family arrive in the hospital, and is a very important time. While practical details may vary a little from one hospital to another, if asked a question about admission of a child the following general points are good ones to bear in mind and include where appropriate:
1. Meet the child and family preferably in 'neutral territory', e.g. admissions department, playroom of ward.
2. Greet them by name, preferably getting down to the level of the child for eye contact. Include parents, siblings and any obvious beloved toy in the welcome, and appear friendly and relaxed.
3. You can pay the child and parents a compliment if appropriate, e.g. on the child's appearance, or comment on journey, to establish a rapport.
4. Show child and his parents to his bed area; leave to unpack and personalize with possessions.
5. Introduce him to other children and parents nearby; take on a brief tour of ward, pointing out important areas, e.g. toilet, bathroom and playroom.
6. Show them where the parent will sleep, if appropriate.
7. It is usually best to let the child stay with the parents during the admission interview. A child who is old enough can answer some of the questions for himself, e.g. name and address, favourite foods, toys, etc.

Besides basic details, important matters to find out about are:
- (a) the name by which the child is usually known
- (b) toilet needs and habits, and words for them
- (c) special toys and comforters, and names of these
- (d) eating habits, e.g. use of cup, spoon, teacher beaker
- (e) special likes and dislikes, especially food and drink
- (f) relations between child, parents and siblings
- (g) developmental progress and special difficulties, especially for the young and handicapped
- (h) personality of child; how he handles stress
- (i) home routines and rituals; family discipline
- (j) schooling or play group if appropriate
- (k) friends, peers
- (l) experience with illness and hospitalization
- (m) preparation for hospitalization
- (n) infectious diseases and immunizations
- (o) cultural and community background.

The interview is best conducted in a quiet, cosy corner of the ward where there should be no interruptions. If there are certain matters which are better not discussed in front of the child, then he could be involved in play with the play leader or other nurses while these are talked about later in the interview.

8. The parents need to be given certain information, e.g. ward name and telephone number; arrangements for being resident and taking meals; visiting times and arrangements; ward routines and how the parents can be involved in caring for the child; when the doctor will see the child, and details of such matters as proposed operation dates and times.

9. A game can be made of putting on the name bracelet so that the child is proud of it, perhaps labelling favourite toy also.

10. Routine observations are best left until last, when the child has settled down. The way in which these are performed may have to be adapted to suit the child (see 3.7 on nursing care), and a game can be made of them, enlisting the co-operation of parents, e.g. weighing mother and child together; taking temperature of teddy.

11. Try to reduce the number of strange events the child encounters soon after coming into hospital, e.g. do not change into night clothes during the day unless essential.

12. Make out care plan based on nursing history; involve parents and older children in planning care when possible.

In an *emergency admission*, although routine information will need to be obtained the priorities are likely to be different. Urgent medical and nursing care may have to be carried out first. Because of the anxieties created by the situation, and the lack of advance preparation, it is even more important for nurses to appear calm, welcoming and reassuring. Appropriate good explanations will have to be given to both child and parents to allay fears.

During the rest of the child's hospital stay, the quality of care he receives, principally from the nursing staff, is vitally important in minimizing the adverse effects of hospitalization.

To summarize the particular concerns and common reactions of children of different ages on coming into hospital:

Age group	Particular concerns	Common reactions
1. Birth – 6 months	(a) Interruption of mother-child bonding process (b) Sensory-motor deprivation	Disruption of developing trust of baby in mother At 4 to 6 months, reacts by crying on separation
2. 6–12 months	Separation – infant recognizes mother as an important person who belongs to him	Anxiety, clinging and crying on separation
3. 1–3 years	(a) Separation – has an intense relationship with mother (b) Change in routines and rituals, so loses sense of security (c) Loss of developing autonomy and independence (d) Loss of mobility (e) Does not fully understand own body, so is fearful of any assault on it	A sequence of reactions if separation is prolonged and not compensated for: (i) Protest – cries, calls out, rejects attention of nurses (ii) Despair – looks sad and apathetic, cries at intervals, sucks thumb or clutches comforter, refuses to eat (iii) Denial – does not react to mother, is more attached to nurses but goes from one to another in quick succession. Accepts care without protest. On

Age group	Particular concerns	Common reactions
		the surface it may seem that he has 'settled down'
		(iv) Regression – to an earlier stage of development. In long-term – may find it difficult to form lasting relationships. With good care, these later stages should not occur
4. 3–5 years	As for 1- to 3-year-old; also, is beginning to have fantasies – may think that parents have abandoned him in hospital as a punishment for some misdeed	As for 1 to 3-year-old; regression is common. Ability to project his feelings on to other people or objects may give rise to aggression – usually physical, sometimes verbal; feelings may be expressed through play or art
5. 5–12 years	(a) Separation – not only from family, but also from schoolfriends (b) Worry about modesty and privacy (c) Anxieties about what is happening to his body; how illness arose (d) Restrictions on mobility	(i) May regress or else attempt to behave in mature fashion (ii) Repress or deny symptoms (iii) Depression (iv) Often develops obsessions and compulsive behaviour (v) Displays phobic anxieties about needles, x-rays, operations, the dark, death, etc
6. Adolescent	(a) Separation from peers and school (b) Worry about how illness will affect	(i) Anxiety and embarrassment (ii) May become angry

Age group	Particular concerns	Common reactions
	body image and sexuality	and reject treatment, denying the need for it
	(c) Lack of privacy and exposure	(iii) May intellectualize to cover up real concerns
		(iv) Depression and withdrawal
		(v) Regression and showing undue dependence on staff or parents

It can be seen from the above chart that the most vulnerable age group in terms of hospital admission and separation from family is from 6 months to 5 years old. Wherever possible, admission in this age group is avoided, but nevertheless, there will be many children in this category in hospital, and they will need particular care and thought.

To meet the needs of children in hospital, the nurse needs not only to be a physical care-giver, but also:
a truthful guardian
a consistent friend
dependable for security
a guide to the environment and treatment procedures
a close observer
a link with the family.

Ideally, the nurse will be accomplishing this in partnership with the child's family, so that the ties within the family are maintained and strengthened. All hospitalized children need the reliable presence of someone important to them, and usually this is a parent. Family-centred care also allows for parents to feel useful and confident in the care of their child, instead of hospital staff taking this over and making parents feel guilty. When families have been involved in care in hospital, it usually takes less time for the child to settle down when he returns home.

Family-centred care requires nurses to communicate well with parents and teach them when necessary, so that they know exactly what is expected of them. Families also need emotional support from nursing staff, and opportunities to have a rest and a break from the hospital atmosphere.

Facilities should be provided and offered for one, or sometimes both, parents to stay in the hospital – this is especially important for the under-

5s. However, in certain circumstances, e.g. if there are several other young children in the family, it may be impossible for a parent to stay. They should not be made to feel guilty about this, but encouraged to visit freely.

In addition to the presence of his family, a child needs:

1. 'Total' care from a limited number of nurses, rather than 'task-oriented' care, so that a child gets to know nursing staff well.
2. A suitably stimulating atmosphere with a daily routine.
3. Opportunities to explore and play in a safe environment. This includes provision of facilities for education in the case of an older child.
4. Explanations and communication at a level the child can understand, both verbally, non-verbally, and through play. These should be honest, so that the child can trust the nurse.

These are all ways in which to minimize the adverse effects of hospitalization on children, so that although some reactions can be expected they will not be too severe nor have long-term effects upon the child after his return home. Some practical ways in which these can be achieved are summarized in the next section. Some examination questions ask about general ways of maintaining normal development while in hospital, as discussed above, but other questions dealing with specific children require more details of how this can be translated into practice, as discussed below.

3.7. Nursing care of children of various ages

This section is intended to be a short summary only of important differences to be considered when undertaking various aspects of nursing care for children.

Observations

These are of great importance, since children can deteriorate very rapidly. As young children are unable to tell you how they feel, and even older children may have difficulty in describing and localizing symptoms, the paediatric nurse has to be acutely observant. Even small changes in behaviour, feeding pattern or vital signs may be significant and should be reported. Alterations in behaviour, e.g. quietness and lethargy, often herald an acute illness and are noticeable some time before any change in other observations is apparent.

Concerning recording vital signs:

1. Respirations and pulse. These are best recorded while the child is quiet before he is disturbed to have his temperature taken. The pulse is difficult

to feel in a young child, although it is easier to feel in the temporal region than elsewhere. For this reason, it is more usual to record the apex beat for a baby under the age of one year.

2. Temperature. Hospital policy regarding this varies a little, but fairly commonly:

(a) Rectal temperature recorded under age of 1 year unless there are rectal abnormalities or diarrhoea.

(b) Axillary temperature recorded between ages of 1 year to 5 to 8 years.

(c) Oral temperature for older children provided there is no mental retardation or danger of convulsion.

N.B. (i) Remember the variations in normal temperature between these sites.

(ii) No child should be left unattended with a glass thermometer in place. When answering a question, always detail the site you would choose for recording the temperature, and where appropriate, suggest ways in which you might go about it, e.g. getting mother to hold child on her lap to keep arm still; explaining to child what is to be done, e.g. 'This stick with numbers tells me how hot you are. Can you help me by cooking it under your arm for a few minutes?' demonstrating on doll, and letting child handle equipment first.

3. Blood pressure. Not always taken as it is difficult to obtain a very accurate result, but necessary in some cases. Always use an appropriate cuff size.

4. Weight. A good guide to the state of hydration and health, especially in a baby or small child. Babies weighed naked, before feeding; young children weighed with minimum of clothing. If the child will not sit or stand still, he can be weighed in the mother's lap or arms, and then the mother's weight subtracted.

5. Fluid balance. Difficult to record accurately, especially before children are toilet trained. Usual to estimate urinary and bowel actions from nappies; if accuracy is vital, a urine-collection bag can be utilized. The help of parents can be enlisted to record input and output; older children may enjoy keeping their own chart, perhaps colouring in pictures of drinks, etc.

Obtaining specimens

1. Urine and stool. To collect a urine specimen before a child is toilet trained, a urine-collection bag is applied after cleaning the genitalia. For twenty-four-hour collections, a special bag with tubing attached is used. Frequent checking is necessary to ensure that the bag is still firmly in place

until the specimen is obtained. After children have been toilet-trained, a clean specimen can be obtained after cleansing the genital region. Until approximately the age of 10, a child does not have sufficient sphincter control to enable a true mid-stream specimen to be collected.

In a young child, a stool sample may be obtained from the nappy. When writing an answer to a question which requires a mention of collection of specimens, not only say what you would collect, but how you would go about collecting it.

2. Nose and throat swabs. A second nurse or mother may need to hold the child if he cannot co-operate, and gently open his mouth. It helps to give a simple description, e.g. 'I am just going to tickle your nose/throat with this little stick'; and let the child see the size of the swab first.

3. Blood samples. Children usually fear these most, and need to be told truthfully what is to be done just before the event. The same procedure may be performed on teddy. A nurse should hold the child and comfort him afterwards. Small children, concerned about body integrity, may worry that the rest of their blood and insides will leak out of the puncture site, and usually appreciate a plaster with a face drawn on it, to restore continuity of the body surface. A mother, if squeamish, may not always be the best person to hold the child in this situation!

Feeding and elimination

The type of feeding will depend on the age of the child and what he is used to at home.

For babies, breast-feeding is the most natural, but bottle-feeding is an acceptable alternative if properly carried out. The mother will have worked out her own routine at home, which is best adhered to in hospital if possible. As a general guide to bottle-feeding, the baby requires:

1. 150 ml per kg in twenty-four hours (more for small babies; less for older babies being weaned);

2. three-hourly feeds during the first fortnight, then four-hourly feeds or on demand;

3. feeds during the night are usually omitted by the age of 2 months. Official recommendations suggest weaning at the age of 4 months, when iron stores in the body need replenishing. Savoury foods are best introduced before sweet things, and one new food should be introduced at a time. Weaning is usually completed at about 9 months, and the baby can cope by then with boiled cows' milk and use a teacher beaker. Minced food can be introduced at the age of 1 year when the baby has some teeth, and can then share the family food.

If discussing diet in an answer to a question, give examples of what would be suitable food and drink. Sick children often like treats of food brought in from home, as most complaints are about hospital food!

Toilet training is usually possible by the age of 2 or 2½, when the nervous system is sufficiently developed to enable voluntary control of sphincter muscles. Before then the baby will be in nappies which need frequent changing and care of the skin to prevent nappy rash. Do not forget these important details in an answer! Potties are usually used for small children at first, progressing to the big toilet with a step or trainer seat. Children find bedpans very difficult to use.

Comfort and cleanliness

Babies are usually bathed daily, if their condition permits, in a baby bath or special sink. When they have achieved back control and can sit unsupported for a while, at 6 to 9 months, they can stay in the bath water a little longer to have a splash and play. Bathtime should always be relaxed and opportunities for play and fun exploited.

Older children should never be left alone in the hospital bathroom, but supervision can be discreet. The water should be run for them, with cold water first, and the temperature tested before getting in. If too sick to go to the bathroom, a blanket bath will be required, and the mother can help or carry this out. Do not forget details of other aspects of hygiene for children, such as combing hair, supervising tooth-cleaning after meals, and hand-washing before meals and after using the toilet. Children do not automatically do these for themselves! Children are usually interested in their clothing, and most prefer to wear their own clothes in hospital. Generally, only very sick children remain in nightwear during the day in hospital. Children like to be allowed to choose clothes to wear, with guidance, especially if wearing hospital clothing.

Play

This is a very important activity for all children, and should never be forgotten in an answer on the care of children in hospital. It is not usually sufficient just to mention that play would be provided, but details of suitable types of play and toys should be given. This will depend on the age of the child (mental age as well as physical age); the presence of any handicaps; and the nature of the illness.

Play in hospital has many objectives and benefits:
1. Allows a child to express his feelings and anxieties, especially in the

strange surroundings of a hospital ward, helping him to come to terms with it.

2. Promotes physical and emotional development; helps to prevent regression during hospitalization; shortens recovery time.

3. Can be used as a means of explaining tests and procedures, e.g. preoperative preparation, to a child.

4. Occupies the child and distracts him from pain.

5. Can compensate for lost abilities, e.g. glove puppets exercise arms and compensate in part for immobility in bed.

6. Can be used in remedial therapy, e.g. blowing bubbles is a useful and entertaining way of doing deep-breathing exercises.

There are various sorts of play, and children need to experience each type of play at some stage to promote proper development. Most play activities are a combination of the different types of play, which are:

exploratory
energetic
skilful
social
creative
problem-solving
hobbies or leisure pursuits (for adolescents and adults).

Children undertake their play in various stages, depending on age, development and ability. The usual pattern is:

1. *Solitary play*: Birth to 2 years. Child plays alone for short periods of time, with an adult in the background.

2. *Parallel play*: 2 to 3 years. Child plays alongside other children but interacts only briefly with them.

3. *Social play*: 3 to 4 years upwards. Child begins to play with others, at first in pairs or small groups. Starts to share toys. Gradually uses all stages of play and interacts with bigger groups.

Handicapped children have special needs for play and play materials, and the help of parents and occupational therapists can be sought to provide suitable play.

Sick children of all ages usually have a very limited concentration span, and so it is necessary to provide a variety of different types of play and play materials, and change them frequently. Most sick children also enjoy passive forms of entertainment, e.g. being told stories, nursery rhymes, having books read to them, listening to the radio and watching television. Some types of play might not be suitable for children with certain conditions, e.g. sand and water play would be inadvisable for a toddler in plaster of Paris. Think carefully before suggesting types of play in an examination answer!

Administration of medicines

All general principles of drug administration apply equally to children, but in addition, the following points should be borne in mind:
1. Two nurses should always be available to check and administer the medicine.
2. Great care should be taken as small dosages are involved and calculations often have to be made.
3. A child's identity should be checked from his name bracelet, not just by asking him his name.
4. Jam or yoghurt, fruit juice and small sweets should be available on the drug trolley to assist in making the medicine more acceptable, or as a reward afterwards.
5. Oral administration is preferable to injections whenever possible.

Guidelines for oral administration of medicines to small children
1. Medicine is best given before feeding, unless contraindicated. A drug should never be put into a feeding bottle or mixed with a meal.
2. A small child should be prepared by being spoken to calmly, and picked up and cuddled if frightened.
3. For a toddler, it may help to let him watch older children co-operating by taking medicines, and by pretending to give teddy some first.
4. One nurse or the parent should hold the child securely while the other administers the medicine.
5. The nurse should be firm that the medicine must be taken, but avoid using force. Care must be taken to ensure that a crying child does not inhale the medicine.
6. Fruit juice or a sweet afterwards helps to take the taste away and promotes co-operation on the next occasion.

Older children generally can co-operate, but may still like a sweet to take away an unpleasant taste. They should sit up to take medicines whenever possible.

Guidelines for giving a child an injection
1. It is essential to be truthful and adequately prepare the child.
2. Two nurses are necessary, one to hold and comfort the child, and one to administer the injection.
3. The injection should be prepared out of sight of the child beforehand.

4. Most children find it difficult to keep still so firm, gentle restraint is necessary to prevent movement of the limb.

5. The child should be comforted immediately afterwards, and an older child praised for his co-operation.

If the child has an intravenous infusion in progress, it might be preferable to use this route for drug administration instead of intramuscular injection. Many children live in fear of when the next 'prick' is coming, no matter how well prepared they are.

Maintaining a safe environment

This is quite difficult in a paediatric ward, which is a hive of activity, and where it is desirable that children have opportunities to move around and explore their environment. Children are not naturally very safety-conscious; rather they are curious and impulsive – so childhood accidents are frequent occurrences. It is the responsibility of nurses to be the eyes and ears for a child, anticipating hazards and taking all possible steps to prevent accidents.

Some potential accidents may be avoided by considering how the child's developmental stage influences the type of accident he is likely to have, e.g. stairs will be a great temptation to a 1-year-old who can crawl, and should be guarded by a gate; hot drinks and saucepans with handles sticking out will be dangerous for a child who has just learnt to pull himself up to standing by holding on to objects.

General measures to maintain a safe environment in a paediatric ward include:

1. Keep children out of certain danger areas, e.g. kitchen, sluice.

2. All drugs, cleaning fluids, urine-testing equipment, etc, to be locked away.

3. No medicines or unnecessary equipment should be left lying around on lockers or trolleys.

4. Put and use gates on stairs.

5. Open doors towards you in case small children are playing behind, unless you can see through the glass.

6. Report any broken items, toys, etc, withdraw from use and have repaired.

7. Use only toys with a B.S.S. kitemark.

8. Do not leave small objects within reach of infant.

9. Turn off electricity at all sockets when not in use; avoid trailing leads on electrical equipment.

10. Mop up all spills on the floor and pick up dropped toys; ensure children wear shoes or slippers when walking around.

11. Keep sharp objects away from children; close nappy pins when not in use.

12. Do not leave children unattended with hot drinks.

13. Cot sides to be raised when small child is unattended, even for a minute.

14. Pillows not used for babies under 1 year because of risk of suffocation.

15. Proper supervision, especially in certain areas, e.g. bathroom, treatment room, playroom.

Any accidents which occur should be promptly reported and investigated. A knowledge of safety factors should be demonstrated in appropriate places in an examination answer.

Pre- and postoperative care

Many aspects are the same as for adults (see Chapter 7 on the management of patients undergoing surgery), but practical details about how the care is achieved in the case of children will vary. Pre- and/or postoperative care is frequently asked about in examination questions on the care of children, so this subject is an important one to revise.

Some special points in the management of children undergoing surgery are:

1. *Preoperatively*:

(a) Emotional support and preparation will be needed both for parents and for child. In the case of the child, it will need to be appropriate to his age, level of development, past experience and degree of understanding.

(b) Find out what the parents and child already know – what preparation has the child received prior to coming into hospital? What does he expect?

(c) Familiarize parents and child with equipment, e.g. operation gowns, masks, anaesthetic apparatus; with location of operating theatres, anaesthetic and recovery rooms; and, if possible, with personnel, e.g. anaesthetist and anaesthetic-room nurse.

(d) Much preparation and familiarization can be achieved in play, e.g. dressing up as surgeons and giving teddy an operation. This allows a child to express his feelings and work out his fears.

(e) Give opportunity for questions, with honest answers.

(f) Prepare child and parents for what to expect postoperatively; both verbally and by demonstrations on dolls.

(g) On the operation day, try to keep a normal routine for as long as possible. Distract the child with play during mealtimes or take him for a bath as he will not be allowed to eat.

(h) Supervise the child to ensure that he is given nothing orally after the appointed time. Because of the risk of hypoglycaemia, small children are usually given a last glucose drink two to three hours before surgery. Explain to parents why he should have nothing orally; a young child may like to select a colourful badge to wear with the message 'Please do not give me food or drink.'

(i) Let the mother help with putting on the operation gown to give her something to do. She could sit and read to the child after he has had his premedication.

(j) Allow the parent to go with the child as far as possible to the theatre; the child's allocated nurse should also go and stay with child until he is anaesthetized. Reassure child, if appropriate, that his mother will be waiting for the child's return to the ward.

2. *Postoperatively*:

(a) Allow the parent to rejoin the child as soon as possible and stay with him to comfort him.

(b) Careful frequent recording of vital signs – children deteriorate very quickly.

(c) Recovery from surgery is usually more rapid than that for adults, and generally less pain is experienced – but do not assume that the child will have no pain. Administer analgesia if required.

(d) Appropriate play activities to distract child as soon as he is able.

(e) Allow the child a chance to talk about his operation and act out his feelings in play.

(f) Give the parents emotional support and necessary teaching in preparation for discharge.

3.8. Discharge of children

If the child is to be discharged from the ward, preparation for this should begin early. (The average length of stay of a child in hospital is now only three days.) It should include:

1. Teaching the child and parents any procedures to be carried on at home.

2. Informing and liaising with family health visitor; district nurse is occasionally required.

3. Telling the parents how much activity the child can undertake at home.

4. Giving specific written advice in certain cases, e.g. after a head injury; after application of plaster of Paris.
5. Making follow-up appointments.
6. Warning the parents about the likely behaviour of the child after return home from hospital. This may take the form of regression; anxious, clinging behaviour; weepiness; naughtiness and wanting own way; quietness and withdrawal

Provided that the child has received good care in hospital, and has opportunities to act out his feelings in play at home with understanding parents, he usually returns to normal after a few days at home. Prolonged disturbance generally indicates that the child's needs have not been adequately met in hospital.

3.9. Specimen R.G.N. questions

Q.1. Identify the essential needs of a four-year-old child and discuss the role of the ward team in the promotion and maintenance of normal development during a period of hospitalization.   100%

English and Welsh National Board, September 1983
R.G.N. Final Examination

Q.2. 'Family involvement in the delivery of care is essential in any paediatric ward.'

Discuss the implication of this statement for:

(a) the sick child and the family   65%

(b) the ward nursing staff   35%

English and Welsh National Board, November 1984
R.G.N. Final Examination

3.10. Sample question and answer

John, aged 6, is being admitted to hospital for adeno-tonsillectomy. He is an only child, and his mother is to be resident with him in the hospital.

(a) Once the admission procedure is complete, describe how nursing staff can prepare John for what is to happen to him.   60%

(b) What are the needs of John's mother during his hospital stay?

                    40%

(*a*) The examiner is trying to find out if you understand the worries and anxieties of a 6-year-old having an operation and if you can relate these to John's needs. It is not enough to say *what* you would tell or do for John; rather, the answer should contain details of *how* you would achieve this.

The sort of details that should be included are:

1. Preparation to be undertaken chiefly by the same nurse who admitted and has been allocated to John as she will have started to build up a rapport with his mother.

2. How has his mother prepared him for the operation?

3. John's understanding of the operation, e.g. Where are his tonsils? What does he think is going to happen? Build upon his ideas and correct misconceptions.

4. Explanation about the operation with John and his mother present.

5. Help to dispel his fear of mutilation by explaining how the tonsils have done their job and are no longer required, emphasizing the aspects of healing and repair, to make John better afterwards.

6. Preparation relating to premedication and anaesthesia:

(a) Invite anaesthetic nurse to meet John so he will see a familiar face next day. Show him theatre gowns and masks.

(b) Allow him to play with a syringe and practise giving an injection to his favourite animal (teddy).

(c) Allow John to play with a box of 'hospital equipment' and act out what is to happen with other children under the direction of the nurse or playleader using dolls and each other.

(d) Identify areas of anxiety by listening to his 'hospital play' and help John discuss these afterwards, as necessary.

(e) Differentiate between 'normal sleep' and 'special or magic sleep' due to anaesthesia.

(f) Ensure John knows he will wake up and reinforce this by discussing his return to the ward and his mother being there when he wakes up. Also, if possible, that his daddy will come and see him later.

7. Preparation for postoperative care by practising lying in a post-tonsillectomy position to enable him to see how this allows saliva to dribble out easily from his mouth. Explain about his sore throat and the medications to make it better and the prospect of his favourite long cool drinks to help his throat get well again soon.

8. Check his understanding by asking him to tell teddy or his favourite toy what is going to happen.

9. His expectation of going home afterwards, e.g. to tell classmates and teachers about the operation. Special present from parents.

(b) The examiner is looking for evidence of an ability to look after not just the child but the mother too, an awareness of her feelings and fears and an understanding of family-centred care.

The sort of details that should be included are:

1. The mother's anxiety as John is an only child and may not have been in hospital before. She needs reassurance, candid explanations and support. This can be provided by trusting relationships with the ward sister and John's key nurse. The staff must take time to chat to her and her husband and give clear descriptions of what is to happen and the approximate timing of events. Her anxiety is likely to be greatest at the time of the operation and it could be suggested that she go out shopping or for a meal with her husband to take her mind off the operation.

2. Involve her in John's care as much as possible, e.g. bathing him, cuddling him, comforting him during his premedication, amusing him with stories and quiet games.

3. Explain to her what to expect postoperatively, e.g. that he will be drowsy, pale and possibly bleed a little from the mouth. The need for frequent observations needs to be explained so she does not feel something has gone wrong.

4. John's mother has physical needs: a comfortable bed, privacy, facilities for having meals and a place to relax.

5. She needs to be given information before discharge to enable her to care for John at home. This should include keeping him at home for a week, away from school and crowded places for two weeks to avoid infection, feeding him a normal diet to encourage healing, and the date of his outpatient appointment.

3.11. Multiple choice questions

Q.1. You would normally expect an infant to reach the milestone of being able to sit unsupported for several minutes at the age of:

(a) *3 months*
(b) *6 months*
(c) *9 months*
(d) *12 months.*

The correct answer is (c); an infant of 3 months is only just starting to have head control; at 6 months he can sit, but only with support; if the infant cannot do this until 12 months, his physical development is delayed, since by then he should be able to stand momentarily on his own.

Q.2. Which of the following would be an unreasonable expectation? That:
(a) *Joe, aged 18 months, can point to his nose and tummy*
(b) *Paul, aged 4, can name colours in a painting*
(c) *Susan, aged 2, can build a tower of six cubes*
(d) *Jane, aged 3, can get herself undressed.*

The correct answer is (d). The other three children should normally be able to accomplish these things at the ages stated. However, Jane, from the age of about 2 will be able to help actively with dressing and undressing, but will not be able to manipulate buttons and accomplish this for herself until approximately 4 to 5 years.

Q.3. A suitable amusement for Stephen, aged 16 months, who is confined to his cot in traction, would be:
(a) *Teething-ring*
(b) *Hammer and peg toy*
(c) *Push-pull musical toy*
(d) *Telling a fairy-tale.*

The correct answer is (b). Children of this age usually enjoy this toy, and it would give him opportunity to use his hands and release pent-up energy, compensating for enforced immobility when normally he would be starting to walk alone. Although at the same age (c) is usually a favourite, it would be unkind to give it to him as he has to remain in his cot. He is rather old for (a), which is normally popular at 6 to 9 months. He is too young, with too short an attention span, for (d), which is usually appreciated by children at about 3 years old.

Q.4. The most effective way of reassuring a toddler being admitted to hospital is to:
(a) Permit his mother to stay with him
(b) Pick him up and cuddle him
(c) Distract him with cuddly toys and sweets
(d) Introduce him to the surrounding children.

The correct answer is (a). This is the most vital factor in reassuring a child in this vulnerable age group; (b) can also be done when necessary, but is of only secondary importance to (a). (c) may be needed in certain circumstances, e.g. if the mother goes out temporarily, but it is difficult to compensate for the absence of the mother. In the case of (d), although this should be done, a toddler will not derive much reassurance from it as he will be far more concerned with himself, and other children will be of lesser interest.

4. Community care

4.1. Introduction

The purpose of this chapter is to summarize the key functions of the primary health care workers and to show how they liaise and interrelate with each other.

Short notes are also included in relation to statutory and voluntary organizations as well as a checklist of agencies to be considered when planning care for patients and clients in the community.

Many questions ask you to *plan for discharge* or *identify agencies that can support that patient/family at home*. The contents of this chapter are appropriate for this type of question.

If you choose to answer a detailed question (e.g. 100 per cent) on the role of the primary health care team, then these notes can only form a basis for your answer and you should need to expand on them from your knowledge and experience.

When answering questions specifically about community care and/or health education in the community, it is important to refer to current reports and research where appropriate. If a health education question is asked it will usually be about subjects which you should be familiar with and are of current interest to both the public and health workers. A list of possible topics is included at the end of the chapter and you are advised to read about them in current nursing and other journals.

It may be that candidates will find that the longer question in the internally set examinations during the transition phase may relate to health education/primary care and family structure as this would reflect the shift in emphasis of the guidelines from the English and Welsh National Board, appropriate to the current syllabus of training.

4.2. *Primary health care workers*

Many people are involved in primary health care and support for patients
and clients in the community. The diagram opposite represents the major
contributors. Those in the inner circle are normally health-centre based
and form the core professional support known as the primary health care
team. Those in the outer circle reflect the most frequently involved
agencies, professional and otherwise, who may be included in the team of
primary health care workers.

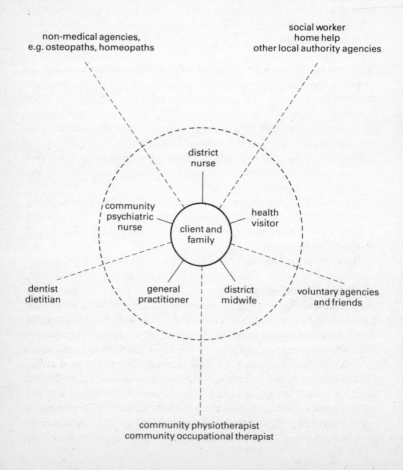

Primary health care team

This term is normally reserved for referring to those *professional* health workers who provide primary care for clients and patients and would always include:
general practitioner
district nurse
health visitor
district midwife
community psychiatric nurse.
Social workers and other community therapists may also be included depending on their specific role in relation to the individual patient.

Some members are predominantly involved in support while others are chiefly involved in prevention of illness.

There are three types of preventive care:
1. *Primary* which is directed towards prevention of illness and includes screening and well-woman clinics.
2. *Secondary* which is directed towards minimizing the effects of illness as a result of early detection.
3. *Tertiary* which is directed towards those who have residual effects from their illness and require support and rehabilitation.

Members of the primary health care team are also involved in health education and this involves:
1. the individual patients
2. the families of the patients
3. other workers – professional or otherwise
4. children in schools
5. students in colleges
6. members of the community in general.

Co-ordination and liaison
The primary health care team, apart from liaising with each other, also liaise with other professional and voluntary workers and will involve family, friends and neighbours in the care of patients where appropriate. They will also need to communicate with hospital workers, ambulance services, police, courts and other statutory agencies as the need arises. They must have a good knowledge of local facilities so as to offer the best service to their clients. They must be familiar with the procedures and policies of the health authorities and advise their clients appropriately.

Some members of the primary health care team have developed special-ist roles within their sphere of responsibility, e.g. an expertise in helping disturbed adolescents, drug abusers, cancer sufferers or other specific client groups. They may undertake training to gain specialist qualifications in, for example, family therapy.

They liaise with the community mental handicap team where necessary, e.g. in dealing with families with handicapped children or caring for handicapped adults.

Health visitor

Health visitors have a unique position among members of the primary health care team as they visit clients routinely and not only if a need has already been identified. This enables them to be in an ideal position for using their skills in the fields of prevention of illness and promotion of health.

The health visitor's work can be categorized in a number of ways, and *all* health visitors are not equally involved with *all* client groups as many have developed a specialized area of interest on which they may concentrate their work.

One type of classification of health visitor is by care groups:
1. Antenatal and postnatal mothers
2. Children 10th day to 5 years
3. Children 5 to 16 years
4. Adults 16 to 65 years
5. Adults 65 years plus
6. Specific client groups
7. Specific health education groups.

Key points relating to care groups
1. *Antenatal and postnatal mothers.* This includes home visiting; baby clinics – which includes developmental screening, advice on minor problems and weighing; advice relating to pregnancy.
2. *Children 10 days to 5 years.* These children are divided into two categories – those who are visited routinely and those who are 'at risk'. The children could be on an 'at risk' register as a result of concern for their mental, physical or social wellbeing.

Children can either be seen in health centres or clinics, or visited at home and advice is given to parents about feeding, immunization and general care.

The health visitor is also able to observe children for developmental milestones and can thus identify at an early stage if normal physical or emotional development is slow or not taking place. The health visitor, in conjunction with other members of the community handicap team, offers support to parents with physically or mentally handicapped children.

She is also in a position to identify other family problems and needs and can initiate action, provide support herself or make appropriate referrals, e.g. marital therapy or housing needs.

3. *Children 5 to 16 years.* This client group is at school and the health visitor therefore can direct her care towards health education and promotion of health in the school situation. It involves work with the school nurse in relation to medicals and immunizations and also work as an educator in the form of classroom lectures and discussions relating to the promotion of health.

The health visitor must still maintain support and involvement with families especially where problems are identified in relation to school attendance. Involvement is also continued with those families where there are handicapped children.

4. *Adults 16 to 65 years.* Visits to this client group can be in connection with, for example, following up cervical smear defaulters; sexually-trans-mitted-disease contacts; any family-related problems; financial problems; marital problems; social problems; physical and mental problems where the involvement of a health visitor is deemed to be appropriate by the primary health care team in addition to, or instead of, the district nurse or community psychiatric nurse.

5. *Adults 65 years plus.* This client group would be visited for reasons as above. In addition, some elderly clients are classified as 'at risk' and the health visitor would be involved with this group specifically.

6. *Specific client groups.* These may reflect the health visitor's specific interest areas or be related to the type of clients in her catchment area, e.g. problem families; single-parent families; immigrant families; adolescents; drug dependents.

7. *Specific health education groups*, e.g. antenatal; mother and children; parent support; solvent abuse; elderly; obesity.

The health visitor is predominantly involved in promotion of health and prevention of illness and for many health visitors much of this work involves families with young children.

The key agencies that health visitors are involved with can be seen on p. 70.

Liaison links for health visitor

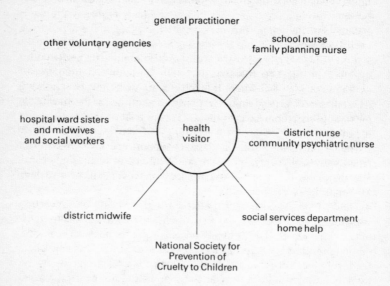

District nurse

The district nurse is involved in providing skilled nursing care to patients in their own homes. She may often have other professionals working under her, e.g. staff nurse, enrolled nurse, as well as nursing auxiliaries. The district nurse is responsible for assessing nursing needs, prescribing care and evaluating the effectiveness of the care given. She may often have to delegate this care to other members of her team or to patients and relatives.

Although the district nurse is involved mostly with caring for patients with an established illness or physical problem she can still be involved in health education with the patients and families she visits.

Her patients can include those requiring care relating to:
early discharge or 'day case' surgery
major hospital surgery
medical illnesses requiring hospital treatment
medical illnesses not requiring hospital treatment
chronic physical disablement

specific conditions, where without support the patient could not remain in the community, e.g. diabetics who are unable to administer their own insulin
terminal care and support.

District nurses can be based in surgeries of general practitioners, health centres or clinics. In these situations they may also be involved in other aspects of primary care work, e.g. immunization administration; first-aid clinics; 'ulcer' clinics; counselling in relation to specific interest areas, such as bereavement, coping with chronic illness; screening, as in carrying out electrocardiographs on 'at risk' patients.

The district nurses' role complements the role of the ward sister in hospital, but it also requires a high degree of involvement with other agencies on a personal level. The district nurse needs to be familiar with the way in which she can obtain aids for her patients and with when to involve other agencies.

The types of agencies she is involved with are illustrated.

Liaison links for district nurse

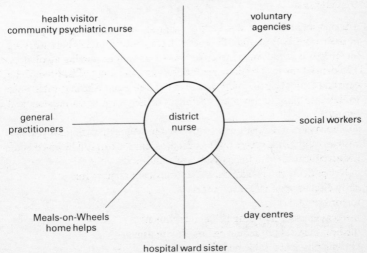

Community psychiatric nurse

Community psychiatric nurses are involved in all levels of preventive care. Many are now health-centre- as opposed to hospital-based and there is an increasing emphasis on their operating under an 'open' referral system.

Key points of the role of the community psychiatric nurse
1. Provision of psychiatric nursing care to clients in the community, e.g. administration of prescribed medication; assessment, delivery and evaluation of care; counselling and listening.
2. Provision of therapeutic activities and treatments, e.g. behaviour therapy; psychotherapy.
3. Acting as a resource to other members of the primary health care team for advice and information about psychiatric nursing care requirements for clients.
4. Education of members of the public and other professionals about mental health and the effects of disorder.
5. Involvement in health education programmes in schools, health centres and community facilities.
6. Support of patients following discharge from hospital.
7. Liaison and co-operation with other agencies.

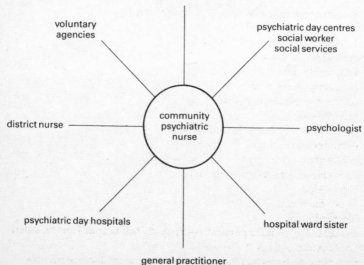

Liason links for community psychiatric nurse

4.3. Statutory and voluntary organizations

Statutory services are those which are funded by central or local government and do not depend on charitable contributions.

Voluntary services are dependent on charitable contributions although they may also receive grants from local or central government.

Although funded differently these agencies should be considered together when planning care for patients and clients in the community. Often there are very strong links between primary health care team workers and social services with voluntary agencies to provide a service for clients they are unable to provide themselves.

It is impossible to list all the organizations involved and the following is only a representative selection. You should supplement this with your own local knowledge of the agencies and facilities with which you are familiar.

Facilities relating to children are discussed in greater detail in Chapter 3.

Statutory services available in the community

1. Health service provision includes:
general practitioner
community district nurse
community district midwife
community psychiatric nurse
health visitor
hospital doctors, nurses, social workers
other paramedical staff
family planning services.
2. Social services provision includes:
home helps
Meals-on-Wheels
luncheon clubs
day centres, e.g. for the physically or mentally handicapped and the elderly
holidays and outings
reductions on buses and trains for elderly and some disabled persons

residential care for children and the elderly
specific services for children in relation to the Child Care Act 1980
day nurses
registration of child minders
supervision orders for young persons under 17 years of age.
3. The probation service.
4. Environmental health inspector.
5. Local authority housing.
6. Department of Health and Social Security benefits include:
(a) *Contributory benefits*:
maternity
sickness
invalidity
unemployment
widow's pension
retirement pension
death grant.
(b) *Non-contributory benefits*:
child
supplementary
industrial injury
mobility and attendance allowance.

Voluntary agencies in the community

These include
Red Cross and St John's Ambulance Brigade
National Society for Prevention of Cruelty to Children (N.S.P.C.C.)
Women's Royal Voluntary Service (W.R.V.S.)
Central Council for the Disabled
Citizen's Advice Bureau
housing associations
marriage guidance services
Age Concern/Help the Aged
church organizations
The Samaritans
organizations involved with specific mental and physical handicap groups,
e.g. Spinal Injuries Association; M.I.N.D.; National Association for the
Deaf, Blind and Rubella Handicapped
agencies involved with addiction problems
support groups, e.g. Asthma Society; Leukaemia Society; Coeliac Society

agencies involved with family planning and childbirth
associations involved with emotional, sexual and developmental problems
health education organizations.

4.4. Health education

Health education should be carried out by all nurses whether working in
a community or hospital setting. It is an important part of the care a
patient receives while in hospital or the community, and should include
such matters as, for example, education about diet to obese and overweight
patients; education about lifestyle to patients suffering from stress-related
illnesses.

It is also important that health education is directed at people who do
not have existing illness or those who if they continue their present lifestyle
are at risk of developing problems associated with their poor health
practice. It is in these fields that members of the primary health care team
are predominantly involved.

In answering a question relating to a specific health-education topic the
following should be considered:
1. Identification of the issues involved.
2. Why is there poor health practice or a need for education?
3. Who is the education directed at?
4. The role of the health educator in providing help.
5. Problems occurring as a result of poor health practice.
6. Other agencies from whom help can be sought.

These points can be illustrated by considering what should be included
in an essay question.

For example,

Q. Discuss the points that should be included by a community nurse
when presenting a session on alcohol abuse to the public at her local
health centre.
1. *Identification of issues*
(a) What is 'normal' drinking?
(b) What is abuse?
(c) Give examples and discuss different drinking patterns
2. *Why is there poor health practice?*
Causes of alcohol abuse, e.g. peer-group pressure; learned from parents;
reduces tension; decreases inhibition; casual drinking progressing to
dependence; dependent personality-type.

3. *Who is the education directed at?*

(a) Those 'drinkers' at risk

(b) People with an established problem

(c) Children/young adults.

4. *The role of the health educator*

(a) Providing information/support

(b) Referral to appropriate agencies

(c) Counselling about effects on health

(d) Organizing group discussions/activities

(e) Involving family and friends

(f) Education of parents about signs of abuse to look for in children.

5. *Problems occurring as a result of poor health practice*

(a) Affects foetal health in pregnancy

(b) Causes physical ill health, e.g. liver cirrhosis

(c) Can cause mental ill health

(d) Affects family life/relationships

(e) Affects work performance

(f) Associated with accidents/anti-social behaviour.

6. *Other agencies from whom help can be sought*

(a) Alcoholics Anonymous

(b) Local support groups and/or counselling services.

Health education topics

The following list is meant as a guide to students as to the type of subjects which should be included when revising this area of the syllabus. The importance of reading current articles and research cannot be overstressed in relation to health education issues as it is vital for the nurse to be up to date with the latest ideas and theories so that she can offer the best advice to patients.

alcohol
breast-feeding
cancer control
child care and development
dental health
family planning
heart disease
lifting
nutrition
retirement
sex education

sexually transmitted diseases
slimming
solvent/drug abuse
stress and relaxation
smoking
vaccination/immunization.

5. Care of patients with psychiatric problems

5.1. Introduction 5.2. Psychological theories: behavioural; psychoanalytical; phenomenological 5.3. Key words 5.4. Psychiatric disorders 5.5. Drugs; antidepressants; anxiolytics; anti-psychotic drugs 5.6. Sample question and answer 5.7. Multiple choice questions

5.1. Introduction

This chapter includes a summary of the different psychological theories, definitions of key words used in psychology and psychiatry and the main general characteristics associated with major psychiatric disorders which the general nurse may encounter when caring for patients with the illnesses in the general ward or department. Brief notes on the common drugs used in treating psychiatric disorders are also included.

As a result of your psychiatric nursing experience, it is expected that you will have a better understanding of the psychological needs of patients admitted to general wards for physical treatment, who also have a psychiatric illness.

It is also expected that you will be able to recognize common signs of mental disorder in patients who are being treated for physical problems and seek appropriate guidance where necessary.

Examination questions relating specifically to the care of patients with a psychiatric disorder are usually presented as either/or questions. The other common presentation is as part of a question which includes aspects of general nursing care and management. For example,

Q. Mary Brand, 22 years old, has been treated by her general practitioner for depression since the breakdown of her marriage eight months ago. She has been admitted to the medical unit after taking a large quantity of tricyclic antidepressant tablets. On admission she is conscious but very drowsy and uncooperative.

(a) Outline the general features of depressive illness.   40%

(b) Describe the specific nursing care Mary will need during her first forty-eight hours in hospital.   60%

Final R.G.N. paper, General Nursing Council for England and Wales, March 1983

5.2. Psychological theories

There are a number of different approaches to psychology. All of them are ultimately trying to explain why we have developed in the way we have psychologically, and what factors influenced this. Key points in three major approaches are summarized below.

Behavioural approach

Behaviourists are concerned with studying individuals by observing their behaviour rather than being concerned with what happens in their brain. J. B. Watson is considered to be the founder of this particular approach.

A major exponent of the theory was I. Pavlov who developed the theory of *classical conditioning* – whereby a particular response leads to a particular consequence (stimulus–response psychology), e.g. the Rat and Skinner box experiment. Traditional behaviourists were only concerned with observable behaviour, and when applying this to treating patients they considered that the fear of spiders, for example, was merely a conditional emotional reaction and could be changed by a reconditioning programme. Nowadays more interest is taken in the patient's feelings about the problem and the way in which the behaviourist is going to approach treating it.

Psychoanalytical approach

Psychoanalysts are concerned with explaining people's behaviour in terms of unconscious motives. They believe that people repress unacceptable or uncomfortable experiences deep in their unconscious minds and that these unresolved conflicts then fester and come to the surface on occasions as symptoms of psychiatric illness. Freud is usually credited with proposing the basic psychoanalytical theory of development.

The main points of Freud's theory are:
1. Everyone has two basic primitive drives: sex and aggression.
2. Personality consists of three parts:

(a) The *id* responsible for our pleasure-seeking impulses

(b) The *ego* which controls when we can satisfy the id drives

(c) the *superego* which is the 'conscience' and decides whether an action is right or wrong.

3. Personality development has distinct stages:

(a) Oral: first year of life

(b) Anal: second year of life

(c) Phallic: third to sixth year of life

Latency period

(d) Genital: adolescence.

4. We are protected against anxiety by unconscious processes called *mental defence mechanisms*.

The id, ego and superego normally work together to produce a well-adjusted personality. If, however, the desires of the id are in conflict with the ego and the superego, then anxiety results.

Psychoanalysts also believe that if problems are experienced at any of the stages of development then this may be reflected in the type of personality. For example, a person who had problems and conflicts over toilet training during the anal stage may develop an obsessive personality in later life.

There are many other psychoanalytical theorists, many of whom reflect a more modern view that society and culture have just as important an influence on development as instinctual drives.

Phenomenological approach

This approach concentrates on subjective experience. It is concerned with how the individual understands events and with his perception of himself and his external environment. Two important theorists in this area are Carl Rogers and Abraham Maslow.

Rogers's theory is based on a self-concept and he believes that we evaluate every experience in relation to our self-concept. We also have an ideal self which is what we would like to be. If there is a marked conflict between our self-concept and either reality or our ideal self then this leads to anxiety. He believes that we all strive towards self-actualization – total fulfilment of one's potential – and that this is the basic driving force for our motivation.

Maslow also theorized in this area and produced a hierarchy of needs where those at the bottom had at least to be partially satisfied before those higher up became important.

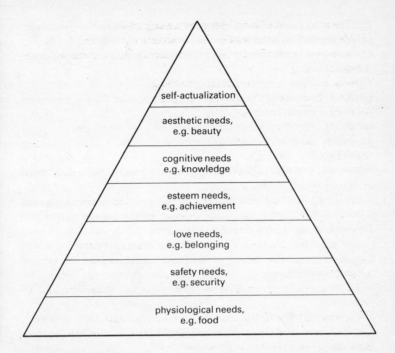

self-actualization

aesthetic needs,
e.g. beauty

cognitive needs
e.g. knowledge

esteem needs,
e.g. achievement

love needs,
e.g. belonging

safety needs,
e.g. security

physiological needs,
e.g. food

5.3. Key words

Abreaction: rapid release of emotion in a psychotherapy session

Affective disorder: prolonged disturbance of mood or emotional feeling state

Anxiety: an apprehensive state where the person has a vague sense of impending danger

Anorexia: loss of appetite

Cognitive disorder: disorder of thought, knowledge or reasoning processes

Delusion: an unrealistic, false belief

Electroconvulsive therapy (E.C.T.): the passing of a small electric current through the brain so as to cause an epileptic-type convulsion

Emotion: a feeling, e.g., anger, joy, which may be associated with slight physiological changes

Endogenous depression: depression caused by deep-rooted unresolved conflicts within the subconscious

Exogenous (reactive) depression: depression caused by life events, e.g. break-up of marriage

Flight of ideas: rapid flow of apparently unrelated ideas in conversation

Group therapy: group discussion/activity with a therapeutic purpose

Hallucination: a false perception for which there is no appropriate external stimulus

Illusion: a misinterpretation of an actual sensation

Intelligence: the ability to interpret experience, learn from it and adapt behaviour appropriately

Libido: the energy of the sexual drive (instinct)

Modelling: the process of learning behaviour by observing and imitating others

Neurosis: a psychiatric disorder in which the patient still retains touch with reality

Personality: the characteristic ways in which an individual thinks and behaves in relation to himself, others and his environment

Psychosis: a psychiatric disorder in which there is a loss of touch with reality and disintegration of personality structure

Thought block: abrupt halting of train of thought or speech followed by preoccupied silence.

5.4. Psychiatric disorders

Psychoses

Psychotic symptoms can be produced as a result of:
1. an underlying psychiatric illness, e.g. schizophrenia
2. abuse of substances, e.g. drugs and glue
3. organic brain damage, e.g. due to dementia.

Key features of psychotic illness

The patient may exhibit some or all of these:
1. personality disintegration/change
2. loss of touch with reality to some extent
3. hallucinations
4. delusions
5. disorders of speech and thought processes
6. irrational/aggressive behaviour
7. social withdrawal/isolation
8. neglect of personal appearance/hygiene.

Key aspects of nursing management
1. Try to establish a trust relationship.
2. Be consistent in your approach.
3. Try to be calm and not raise your voice, even if angry.
4. Don't label the patient as, for example, 'schizophrenic'.
5. Involve him in conversation.
6. Encourage social interaction.
7. Involve family or persons with whom he is familiar in his care if practicable.
8. Appreciate that the patient really does experience hallucinations and believes his delusions to be true.

In most cases it is best not to agree with a patient's delusional ideas or hallucinations, as this reinforces them, and also not to (logically) disagree strongly with them. Adopt an approach wherein you say that you will not discuss them with the patient as they are unrealistic and try only to discuss other topics with him thereby reinforcing realistic ideas.

Neuroses

Neurotic disorders are all of an emotional origin.
    They can be divided into five major groups:
1. Depression
2. Anxiety states
3. Phobias
4. Obsessive-compulsive states
5. Hysterical reactions.
    The most commonly encountered in patients on a general ward is depression and the notes below relate to this only.

Key features of depression
1. Feelings of hopelessness/worthlessness/inadequacy/guilt
2. Loss of libido
3. Loss of appetite
4. General tiredness/lethargy
5. Feeling tearful
6. Exaggerates shortcomings/weaknesses
7. Underestimates achievements
8. Lacks enthusiasm/sparkle
9. May be agitated
10. Sleep disturbances

11. May express suicidal thoughts/intentions
12. Flatness of affect.

Key aspects of nursing management

1. Try to establish a trust relationship.
2. Be consistent in your approach.
3. Reinforce positive attitudes and feelings.
4. Encourage conversation and social interaction.
5. Spend time listening to the patient.
6. Encourage family and/or friends' involvement if possible.
7. Allow patient to talk about feelings and/or precipitating factors.
8. Observe closely but discreetly for suicidal tendencies.
9. Administer antidepressant medication as prescribed.

5.5. Drugs used in treating psychiatric disorders

Antidepressants

'Tricyclic' compounds (and related drugs)
For example, imipramine, amitriptyline.

Key facts
1. Drugs may take two to three weeks before effect is noticed.
2. Remission usually occurs after three to twelve months' treatment.
3. All have a sedating effect (imipramine less than amitriptyline).
4. Cardiac arrhythmias are a serious side effect.
5. Other side effects include dry mouth, blurred vision, constipation, urinary retention and sweating.

It is important to be aware of the side effects when caring for patients who have taken overdoses of these drugs, especially the cardiac effects, and this is why these patients are always admitted to hospital for cardiac monitoring.

Monoamine oxidase inhibitors (M.A.O.I.s)
For example, Nardil, Parnate.

Key facts
1. These drugs have serious drug and dietary interactions.
2. Response to treatment can be immediate but may take three weeks or more.

3. General side effects include postural hypotension and dizziness.
4. Severe *hypertensive* reaction occurs with certain drugs and food.
5. Patients should carry a Treatment Card at all times.
6. Foods to avoid include cheese, pickled herring, Bovril, Oxo, Marmite or other meat or yeast extract, Chianti wine.
7. Alcohol should only be drunk in moderation.
8. The danger of side effects persists for up to two weeks after treatment is stopped.

Anxiolytics

For example, diazepam, lorezepam.

Key facts
1. These drugs are given to reduce anxiety.
2. Tolerance to effects develops within four months.
3. Dependence occurs in susceptible patients.
4. They increase the effect of alcohol.
5. Side effects include sedation, dizziness.

Anti-psychotic drugs

For example, chlorpromazine, haloperidol.

Key facts
1. Used as major tranquillizers
2. Marked sedative effect
3. Effective in reducing psychotic symptoms
4. Side effects are associated with extra-pyramidal symptoms
5. The Parkinsonian effects may be suppressed by giving anticholinergic drugs, e.g. procyclidine
6. Other side effects include hypotension.

5.6. Sample question and answer

Q. Jan Watson, aged 27, is admitted to the accident and emergency department having slashed her wrists in a suicide attempt. She is accompanied by a friend who says she has been depressed following the recent break-up of her marriage.

(*a*) *Describe the nurse's role in the immediate care and treatment which Jane will receive in the Accident and Emergency Department.*   (40%)

(*b*) *What psychosocial information should be obtained during nursing assessments in order to plan Jane's care in hospital and support on discharge?*   (60%)

(*a*) Your answer should include the following:

1. Stop bleeding by application of firm dressing.

2. Elevate arm as required.

3. Observe and record blood pressure, pulse rate, respiratory rate and skin colour for evidence of shock.

4. Assist doctor with:

(a) obtaining a blood specimen for grouping and cross-matching if patient is shocked

(b) administration of anaesthetic

(c) cleaning wound aseptically and suturing.

5. Bandage wrists firmly after suturing and elevate arms.

6. Administer long-acting penicillin, e.g. Triplopen and tetanus toxoid, and analgesia, such as paraveretum if prescribed.

7. Remove any clothing or other possessions, e.g. a knife, which could be used for further suicide attempts.

8. Ensure the safe administration of the blood transfusion if prescribed.

9. Arrange for admission to a ward in the hospital.

10. Remain with Jane at all times.

11. Reassure her and explain to her what is happening.

(*b*) The psychosocial assessment would commence when Jane was admitted to the ward as she would probably be too ill or distressed for it to be effectively conducted in the accident and emergency department, although the friend who accompanied her would be an important source of information. The assessment would be ongoing and depend on a key nurse establishing a relationship of trust with her.

In order to plan her care, information would need to be obtained on:

1. *Social situation*:

Where does she live?

What type of accommodation is it?

Does she have employment?

If so – what? Does she want her employer contacted?

Does she have many friends?

What are her interests/hobbies?

Who is looking after her accommodation while she is in hospital? Friends/neighbours?

2. *Family situation*:

Are there children?
Why did the marriage break up?
Had there been previous problems?
Does she wish her husband to be contacted?
Are her parents alive and well?
Does she have a good relationship with them?
What other family is there, e.g. brothers?

3. *Psychiatric history*:
Has she attempted suicide before?
Is she currently taking any medication and what is it?
Has she ever had previous psychiatric problems?
If so, where was she treated and by whom? For example, visited by community psychiatric nurse; attending a day hospital/outpatients department; as an inpatient.
Does she seem depressed?
What signs of depression is she exhibiting? For example, feelings of worthlessness/guilt; lethargy/tearfulness/flatness of affect; sleeping pattern.

4. *Involvement with other agencies*:
Has the general practitioner seen her recently?
Is a social worker involved with her problems?
Has she had marriage-guidance counselling?

5. *Jane's attitude to being in hospital*:
Her feelings about the incident.
Her expectations about the future.
Her attitude to community support, if appropriate.

5.7. Multiple choice questions

Q.1. Which of the following terms best describes the power of projecting oneself into the feelings of another person or situation?
(*a*) *sympathy*
(*b*) *empathy*
(*c*) *modelling*
(*d*) *identification*.

The correct answer is (*b*).

(c) is learning behaviour by observing and imitating others. (*d*) is the process of acquiring aspects of personality and behaviour from significant people during the developmental years. (In Freudian terminology it is the unconscious mechanism which describes taking on the personality characteristics of someone you have great conflicts about.)

(*a*) is harmonious understanding and compassion involving community of feeling.

Q.2. Which of the following terms correctly describes the process of relegating a psychologically traumatic or conflicting episode into the unconscious mind without the individual being aware of the process?
(*a*) *repression*
(*b*) *regression*
(*c*) *suppression*
(*d*) *substitution.*

(*a*) is the correct answer.

(*b*) refers to reverting to the childhood stage of life. (*c*) is a conscious process of withholding information. (*d*) refers to a defence mechanism whereby emotionally painful experiences are replaced by ones which can be enjoyed.

Q.3. Which of the following states may result from failure to observe dietary precautions when taking monoamine oxidase inhibitor drugs?
(*a*) *an acute hypotensive episode*
(*b*) *a sudden and severe hypertensive episode*
(*c*) *severe anaphylaxis*
(*d*) *depression of respiratory centre.*

The correct answer is (b).

(a) can occur with overdose or in susceptible patients not with dietary indiscretion. (c) and (d) could not result from dietary indiscretion.

Q.4. Which of the following is a characteristic feature of manic-depressive illness?
(*a*) *disturbance of affect*
(*b*) *primary delusions*
(*c*) *thought blocking*
(*d*) *delusional perception.*

(*a*) is the correct answer as this condition is associated with mood swings from depression to elation.

(*b*), (*c*) and (*d*) are generally associated with psychotic disorders like schizophrenia.

6. Care of the elderly person

6.1. Introduction 6.2. The ageing process 6.3. Benefits and facilities available to the elderly 6.4. Pathological conditions associated with old age 6.5. Crisis events of later life 6.6. Nursing problems 6.7. Sample question and answer

6.1. Introduction

Very often in the examination paper you will find that a number of questions relate to current topics of clinical or social interest or concern. One of these topics is care of the elderly person. As the number of people over the age of 65 in the population continues to rise, a much greater proportion of nursing care and resources is directed towards meeting the particular needs of this group of people.

A point that is emphasized in this chapter is that *old age itself is a natural and normal process*: people are not necessarily ill by virtue of being old.

However, the changing physiological, social and psychological status of an old person may, in varying degrees, affect the way in which care is planned, delivered and evaluated even though the specific condition which is being suffered or experienced is one which could happen to a person at any stage in his life. An example of this can be seen in a recent state final examination paper.

Q. Mr Roberts, aged 75 years, is partially sighted and lives in a warden-controlled flat. While shopping he slips on a wet floor, sustaining a Colles fracture.

Describe how the nurse should meet Mr Roberts's needs:

(a) in the Accident and Emergency Department   40%

(b) until he is discharged home 24 hours later   60%

Final R.G.N. paper, English and Welsh National Board, March 1985

A Colles fracture is a mishap which can befall anyone and requires clear-cut medical and nursing intervention. What you must do in this case is decide to what extent Mr Roberts's age, infirmity and social situation should affect the way in which you must plan and deliver nursing care which takes into account all of these factors.

A large section of this chapter is therefore concerned with identifying the features of normal ageing and distinguishing between the normal and abnormal ageing process. We will also consider some pathological conditions which mainly afflict people in later life. In addition, it is necessary to be aware of life-crisis events which are most common in the elderly, and finally to examine certain nursing problems which are frequently encountered when caring for old people either in hospital or in their own homes.

Remember, it is no more possible to generalize about old people than about any other section of the population. The majority of the most powerful people in the world, and many of the most famous and well-loved, have already lived considerably longer than the biblical 'three score years and ten', though conversely we can all think of individuals who strike us as being old and helpless although they may scarcely have reached normal retiring age.

6.2. The ageing process

It is estimated that the absolute potential lifespan of the human being is not more than 120 years, by which time inevitable and irreversible ageing will have overtaken the individual. Ageing is usually considered with regard to the physical, psychological and social changes that occur in the person but it must be borne in mind that these three areas interact and are to some extent interdependent. The onset of perceptible signs of ageing varies very much from person to person but it is the established convention in our society to think of the elderly person as an individual who has passed the age of 65. Ageing happens gradually in most cases and evidence of change in one aspect of life does not necessarily indicate that the other changes are happening at the same rate.

Physical ageing

1. Outward signs:
(a) Changes in hair, skin, sensory acuity
(b) Loss of suppleness and easy mobility; loss of muscle tone.

2. Physiological changes:
(a) Reduction in hormone production affecting secondary sex character-istics; changes in gastrointestinal absorption efficiency and mobility (with implications relating to nutritional needs and elimination problems).
(b) Degenerative processes affecting all the body systems but particularly skeleto-muscular and cardiovascular systems; slowing down of cell repli-cation and tissue repair mechanisms; neurological degeneration which affects sensory perception and response, reflexes and speed of reaction of the body's compensatory mechanisms.

Psychological emotional ageing

1. Increased preoccupation with the past
2. Reduced efficiency of recent as opposed to distant memory
3. Unwillingness and reduced ability to adapt to change
4. Acquisition of new knowledge becomes more difficult and less effective
5. Alterations in emotional state can become more abrupt and profound
6. The circle of acquaintance and experience gradually closes in, leading to a tendency for the old person to be withdrawn and isolated from the world around.
N.B. Many people retain their sexual drive until very late in life and the need for love, affection and appreciation *never* diminishes.

Social ageing

In most cases a change occurs taking the elderly person from an indepen-dent, useful place in society to a dependent, non-productive role. For many people, old age means a transition from comparative comfort to near poverty, leading to a necessary reduction in the amount of social and leisure activity that can be undertaken. For others, however, old age can demonstrate a positive move from a busy, duty-filled life to a state of freedom and opportunity for self-fulfilment.

Loss of status and the feeling of being a burden to family and community is a common experience. The old person in society is often dependent on concessions and privileges in order to maintain an adequate standard of living, e.g. pensioners' reduced rates, extra benefits and allowances, special appeals for the elderly – all of which can impair the self-respect of the individual. You must remember that the social status of the individual can be affected according to the ethnic as well as social group to which he belongs.

The complexity of our society, particularly for those from underprivileged or minority groups, frequently exacerbates problems which can arise from an individual's efforts to come to terms with the changes in his life. Modern society is geared to associate youth with beauty, pleasure and usefulness, and old age with unattractiveness, insensitivity and burdensome dependence and it is this concept which is at the root of a high proportion of the difficulties encountered when caring for elderly people.

Normal versus abnormal ageing

1. Abnormal ageing occurs when the ageing process progresses at a rate which is not catered for by the expectations of the social group to which that person belongs.
2. It also occurs when certain aspects of the process are accelerated especially if other areas of experience are less affected, e.g. intellectual impairment outstripping physical and social ageing as occurs in demented people.
3. A normal ageing process may be directly associated with a pathological condition which thereby makes it disproportionately handicapping, e.g. normal reduction in mobility with severe degenerative joint disease.

The nurse should regard ageing as a problem only if and when the normal processes are creating difficulties for the patient in preventing him from maintaining his independence in carrying out normal daily-living activities.

6.3. Benefits and facilities available to the elderly

This section is intended to enlarge on the comments made about social ageing.

You need to be familiar in principle with the provisions made by the State for the welfare of old people. This is a highly complex arrangement and is constantly changing. One of the best ways of ensuring that you are up to date is to visit your local Department of Health and Social Security (DHSS) office, or better still, if there is one nearby, Age Concern centre, and obtain the pamphlet entitled *Which Benefit* FB2 together with any other available information.

You need to distinguish between entitlements such as:
State pension
free medical and dental services, which should be routinely obtained
Supplementary Benefit and additional allowances, e.g. heating and attendance allowances which need to be applied for. There are also a range of

concessions which apply to old people and which may vary from place to place:
free or cheap travel
reduced prices for theatre or cinema
cheap off-peak holidays.
Welfare facilities may also be available:
lunch clubs
day centres
social centres
domiciliary services, such as chiropody, hairdressing.
These may be organized by:
social services departments
religious groups
professional welfare organizations
charities.

If you feel that the arrangements are complicated, then remember how hard it must be for the potential beneficiary to sort it out.

For further information on this topic you should refer to the chapter on Community Care.

6.4. Pathological conditions specifically associated with old age

In addition to the conditions discussed below you should refer to relevant chapters of the book dealing with:
fractures (particularly femoral); cerebrovascular accidents; heart failure; respiratory disorders; genitourinary problems (prostatic mainly); gynaecological conditions (repairs and hysterectomy); anaemias; diabetes; ophthalmic problems (especially cataracts).

Parkinson's disease

Key facts
1. Disorder of the extra-pyramidal system
2. Associated with a deficiency of the neurotransmitter-dopamine.
3. Can be idiopathic or as a result of drug therapy, e.g. phenothiazines.
4. Important features include uncoordinated and abnormal muscle movements, muscular rigidity, tremors, dribbling, shuffling gait and bent posture with a 'mask-like' expressionless face.

5. The disease is normally progressive, and treatment and care are aimed at slowing down or minimizing the effects.

Key aspects of nursing management
1. Individual care directed at those features of the illness (see above) which cause the patient problems with his activities of daily living, e.g. mobility, feeding, dressing, communicating, enjoying hobbies.
2. Maintaining a safe environment.
3. Showing patience, respect and understanding in order that the patient's frustrations are minimized.
4. Encouraging intellectual pursuits if appropriate as it should not be assumed that intellectual deterioration is present.
5. Administering medical treatment, e.g. levodopa with carbidopa (Sinemet) and observing for side effects.
6. Participating in rehabilitative therapy directed at maintaining the highest degree of independence for the patient within his disability.

Osteoarthritis (degenerative joint disease)

Key facts
1. The commonest joint disease and cause of chronic disability after middle age.
2. A degenerative disease causing, specifically, pain and stiffness.
3. It affects mainly large weight-bearing joints.
N.B. You should be able to draw a joint, e.g. the knee, and illustrate the stages in the progression of degenerative joint disease.

Key aspects of nursing management
Surgical treatment and associated nursing management are discussed in Chapter 13. Care of patients suffering from degenerative joint disease and receiving palliative treatment should emphasize the following factors:
1. Appreciation of patient's handicap
2. Avoidance of strain
3. Pain relief
4. Warmth
5. Assistance in maintaining good posture
6. Gentle exercise and adequate rest
7. Physiotherapy
8. Appropriate mobility aids.

Dementia

Key facts
1. The progressive disintegration of intellect, memory and personality.
2. It is irreversible
3. Memory loss is an early problem – initially forgetfulness, but progressing to global memory deficits about which the patient appears to have no insight.
4. Emotional changes include anxiety, depression, confusion, and suspicion and emotional lability is common.
5. General intellectual decline and fragmentation of the thinking process.
6. Apathy, self-neglect and deterioration in social behaviour.

Key aspects of nursing management
1. A comprehensive nursing assessment of physical and mental health including social situation should be prepared as a basis for planning care.
2. Maximize the patient's remaining abilities.
3. Participate in multidisciplinary approach to provide a simple, stable, structured and stimulating environment.
4. Appropriate care relating to physical problems.

Hypothermia

Key facts
1. A state in which the body temperature has fallen and remains below 35°C.
2. This is not a disease process but it is a common reason for emergency admission of old people to hospital.
3. It should normally be preventable.
4. Causative factors include:
(a) less efficient temperature regulation in the elderly
(b) cold environment, e.g. due to inadequate heating
(c) inadequate clothes
(d) decreased mobility
(e) poor nutrition
(f) loss in insulating subcutaneous fat
(g) underactive thyroid.
Many of these factors are experienced to some extent by a large number of elderly people and once the process starts it is difficult to reverse.

Key aspects of nursing management

1. Assist the patient to regain an adequate body temperature. This must be done gradually on the principle of conservation of existing body-heat production. Too rapid heating may lead to peripheral vasodilatation and profound shock.

2. Restore the patient to an optimum state of physical and mental health.

3. Intravenous rehydration and nutrition may be necessary.

4. Ensure the correction of those factors which contributed to the situation *before* the patient is discharged.

5. Carry out appropriate care for the patient remembering that he or she is likely to be disorientated and confused with little recollection of what has happened.

6.5. *Crisis events of later life*

Retirement

The implications both financial and social will to some extent depend on a person's previous occupation and lifestyle and the way in which he has been prepared for the event. Retirement is a landmark which to many people marks the end of a useful existence. Problems which may arise include: how to occupy time positively; adjusting to new family, especially marital, relationships; how to manage on a reduced income; loss of social contact with colleagues; labelling as 'a pensioner'; increased preoccupation with approaching infirmity.

On the positive side, it must be remembered that for many people, if they have prepared for retirement, this can mark the beginning of a new and welcome stage in life with an opportunity to enjoy leisure and freedom to pursue one's own interests.

Admission to hospital

This may be acute and of short duration or the preliminary to long-term hospitalization. To many old people, going into hospital marks 'the beginning of the end' and may be a deeply distressing experience. There is often a nagging fear that other people will take over and they will never go back to their own homes. It is most important that the patient is treated as a responsible and respect-worthy person who retains the power of personal decision-making. Because adapting to new circumstances is less easy the older one gets, time, patience and gentleness must be expended in orienting the patient to hospital. A full assessment of the patient's total needs must be carried out at the earliest opportunity but care must be taken to avoid a lengthy and what may seem impertinent interrogation.

Most of the nursing staff will be young enough to be the children or grandchildren of the old person. The nurse must make sure she is identifying the patient's needs in relation to his own life experiences and beliefs and *not* those of herself or those which she has arbitrarily decided are appropriate.

Bereavement

By the time a person has reached old age, it is unlikely that he will have failed to experience the loss of a loved one, but this process snowballs with advancing years and it is often the case that one becomes increasingly isolated as family, friends and contemporaries die.

It is very difficult to imagine the effect of the loss of a life partner be it husband, wife, lover or friend, even if the partnership has appeared to an outsider to be unhappy or turbulent. (We should remember at this point that for some people a beloved animal has for years substituted for the companionship of a partner and loss of such a pet is also a form of bereavement.)

In addition to normal grief, bereavement for an old person may give rise to loss of purpose in life; inability to cope alone; depression and fears about his approaching end; problems in coping with the legal and financial aspects of bereavement; a speeding up of the ageing process; and, not uncommonly at this stage of life, suicide. Bear in mind that the more one has had the greater the sense of loss. The nurse must give the bereaved person encouragement to discuss his feelings as well as providing practical support. Many old people conceal their grief. This does not mean they are not experiencing it.

Loss of an independent home

This may happen as a result of reduced financial circumstances or, more frequently, because a person can no longer live independently due to physical or mental infirmity. Loss of one's home is loss of independence especially if it is the environment in which one has spent the majority of one's happy, active and productive years. The accumulation of a lifetime's possessions, with their associated memories and connotations, is centred in the home. It is most important that a person giving up his home has a free choice to select at least some treasured personal possessions which will be treated with the respect that he himself accords them.

There are a number of possible options for a person giving up his home:
1. purpose-built, supervised accommodation, e.g. warden-controlled flat
2. private hotel or rest home
3. living with relatives – usually a child and his or her family
4. private or social-services-run old people's home or nursing home.

These are listed in increasing order of loss of independence and of institutionalization. For many, the obvious choice seems to be for the old person to live with a relative, but this is a commitment which must be considered carefully on both sides, for the tradition of caring lovingly for the aged members of the family within one's own home may be neither practicable in terms of accommodation nor endurable in terms of the social and emotional demands which can conflict with the needs of the son or daughter and their children. The arrangement sometimes works well, in which case it enables the old person to have a happy and fruitful old age as part of the family. This is the ideal solution, but too often a situation arises full of resentment, intolerance and frustration in which love changes to reluctant duty.

If the old person has no alternative to life within an institution, no matter how benevolent it may be, then the onus lies heavily upon the carers to provide a lifestyle in accordance with the right of every human being to a dignified existence incorporating a minimum of dependence.

Approaching death

Death is a topic few people wish to dwell upon and is one of the great taboos of modern society. The older one gets, the more one has to face up to the inevitability of death and this is emphasized as people around one die.

Many old people, especially if they have lived according to a firm religious or philosophical code desire time to think about and prepare for death. The opportunity should never be denied to a person to talk through his feelings, fears and conflicts regarding death (including the arrangements he wants made for his funeral), and the nurse plays an important part in facilitating such expression by, firstly, making time to listen and secondly, by showing that she respects, not only in words but by her attitude, the beliefs and feelings of the person. She must not project her own fears and distaste for the subject by refusing him the right of decent preparation for death. It must also be remembered that although a person may have had a long life, perhaps full of pain and suffering, it must never be assumed that he wants to die or values life less than anyone else.

Often the fear is not of death, but the process of dying in pain and loneliness. The nurse must ensure that as far as is humanly possible, this never happens to a person in her care. The best reassurance any person can have is to see the high quality of care given to other people who are nearer to death than he is.

Many old people will wish to put their affairs in order and arrange the disposal of their possessions. To some people this becomes a fascinating hobby; others use it as a threat to prospective legatees. An old person, as long as he is capable of rational judgement, has a perfect right to spend as much time as he wishes disposing of his goods in his own way and the nurse must beware of being drawn into family conflicts or taking sides.

Approaching death should be regarded as a fact of life and acknowledged in correct relation to each individual's own circumstances and concerns.

6.6. Nursing problems

The following problems are frequently encountered when nursing old people. Under each heading are summarized some key points which will contribute to effective care.

Confusion

1. Ascertain the cause if possible. Is the confusion the cause or result of admission to hospital?
2. Many illnesses lead to confusion, e.g. infections, especially respiratory; cerebral ischaemia due to cardiovascular problems; drug intolerance; constipation.
3. Fear and pain make confusion worse.
4. *Be patient.* Take time to explain and show to the patient those facts and features of the environment which he needs to know. Be prepared to repeat them as often as necessary.
5. Do not overwhelm the person with too much information at any one time.
6. Provide stimuli which help orient the patient to time and place.
7. Encourage the patient to have familiar personal possessions.
8. Keep life simple but dignified.

9. Use appropriate specialized techniques such as Reality Orientation and Reminiscence Therapy.

10. Listen to what the patient is trying to tell you.

Incontinence

1. Is it faecal or urinary or both?

2. Exclude or treat physical causes, e.g. urinary tract infection, constipation, inability to get to the toilet, gynaecological or prostatic disorder.

3. Is the incontinence associated with psychiatric problems, e.g. confusion, depression, dementia?

4. Monitor when, where and how often incontinence occurs.

5. Devise a régime for the patient based on 4 and ensure it is followed. Evaluate and modify as necessary.

6. Always maintain the dignity of the patient.

7. Never withhold or restrict fluids, unless there is a specific medical reason and this is ordered by a doctor.

8. Ensure easy access to sanitary facilities.

9. Never reproach or humiliate a person for his incontinence.

10. Make sensible use of commodes, bedpans, urinals, ensuring privacy for the patient.

11. Make sure the patient is never left on a soiled bed or wearing soiled clothes.

12. Be scrupulous when assisting the patient in his personal hygiene.

13. Use continence aids and garments correctly and economically; remember these will not cure incontinence but may assist in preserving a decent quality of life for the incontinent person.

Pressure sores (*established or high risk*)

1. Remember the contributory causes, e.g. poor nutrition; immobility; incontinence; dehydration; rough handling.

2. Assess patients using the Norton Scale.

3. Ensure that unrelieved pressure on any body surface is never maintained for more than two hours.

4. Help the patient become as physically fit and mobile as possible.

5. Use pressure-relieving devices correctly.

6. Treat every pressure sore as any other wound, using appropriate dressing techniques.

Maintenance of an adequate nutritional state

1. What are the patient's nutritional needs in relation to size, health and activity level?
2. Are there any metabolic problems?
3. Find out what the patient likes to eat and drink and when he normally has his meals.
4. Correct constipation.
5. Ensure oral and dental hygiene.
6. Can the patient physically feed himself and eat the food provided?
7. Use food supplements only if nutrition cannot be achieved.
8. Encourage the patient to drink plenty of the fluids he likes.
9. Try to provide a suitable social environment for meals.
10. Try to help the patient feel life is worth living.
11. Do not give the patient dietary advice which is:
(a) contrary to his own principles, e.g. vegetarian
(b) impractical for him to carry out when he returns home, e.g. too expensive, difficulty in shopping, preparation, cooking.

Rehabilitation

1. The aim of all nursing care must be to enable the patient to regain the optimum level of independence.
2. Rehabilitation is a team programme.
3. Endeavour to motivate the patient.
4. Set realistic goals.
5. Relate as far as possible to the patient's own social standards and environment.
6. Ensure that adequate support services can be provided where necessary.
7. Progress slowly and steadily; evaluate frequently and regularly.
8. Only accurate assessment with ongoing review will enable you to recognize the patient's potential.

6.7. Sample question and answer

Q. Mrs Priest, a slightly confused 84-year-old lady, is admitted to your ward from home as her daughter is no longer able to look after her. She has recently become incontinent of faeces and has been unable to get up from her bed. Her appetite is poor and she is reluctant to drink.

Using a problem-solving approach describe the role of the nurse in prevention of pressure sores based on information obtained during the nursing assessment.   100%

The main problems which can be identified are:
1. Lack of mobility as she is confined to bed.
2. Poor appetite – she is probably already thin and her skin may be in a poor condition.
3. Reluctance to drink – this could lead to dehydration and an increase in her confusion.
4. Faecal incontinence means that there is a risk of skin damage from soiling.
5. Confusion may make it difficult for her to understand or participate actively in her care.
6. Potential disease process or pathological condition may be present which necessitates her remaining in bed.
N.B. The problems you identify and the nursing action *must* relate to the prevention of pressure sores as this is the aspect of care the question is asking about.

Action:
Problem 1:
(a) Carry out a full assessment on admission using all your observational skills.
(b) Assess the risk level of the patient using the Norton Scale or similar and relate the score to your care plan.
(c) Use a variety of techniques to reduce the effects of pressure and shearing forces: frequent and regular change of position; careful and gentle handling and moving; crease-free clothes and linen; use of aids.
(d) Observe, record and report any changes in skin colour or integrity.
(e) Regularly evaluate your care and adjust plan accordingly.
Problem 2:
(a) Be aware of the danger of further weight loss and monitor weight.
(b) Try to find out what the patient likes to eat and provide small, attractive meals of high nutritional value.
(c) Ensure that Mrs Priest has a clean, fresh mouth and that her dentures (if she has any) are well fitting and are worn by her.
(d) Make sure that she is comfortable at mealtimes and give assistance and encouragement.
Problem 3:
(a) Provide plenty of fluids (preferably nutritious) of the kind she likes,

bearing in mind her preference for temperature, sweetness, amounts of milk.

(b) If she can help herself, ensure that a drink is always within reach.

(c) Remind and assist her to drink.

(d) Observe her skin texture and for other signs of dehydration.

(e) Monitor and record fluid intake and urinary output.

Problem 4:

(a) Offer the commode on a regular basis and try to re-establish regular bowel action.

(b) If incontinence occurs do not reproach her, wash and gently dry soiled skin and apply barrier cream.

(c) Change soiled clothes or linen immediately.

(d) Check that she is not suffering from faecal impaction and overflow. If this is so, take appropriate measures to rectify it.

(e) Monitor and record when incontinence occurs.

Problem 5:

(a) Try to encourage her co-operation by showing patience, explain always what is being done and why.

(b) Praise her and show appreciation of her efforts.

(c) Remember that Mrs Priest may find it difficult to express her own needs and may not complain of pain or discomfort. Therefore, your observation and anticipation of needs must be particularly acute.

(d) Do not reinforce her confusion but ensure that you continually and unobtrusively stimulate and orient her to her surroundings.

Problem 6:

As we have no specific information we must simply bear in mind that her risk of pressure sores or prolonged immobility could be increased if she is suffering from a disease, paralysis or any other condition which limits mobility.

7. Management of patients undergoing surgery

7.1. Introduction

The aim of this chapter is to cover those aspects of nursing care which
can be applied to most surgical patients. It includes checklists of points
to remember when planning care both in the pre- and postoperative
phases. Some notes are also included on care in the recovery room and
asepsis. Specific nursing care is included in the relevant later chapters.

The type of questions you will be asked are likely to relate to a specific
aspect of surgical nursing management rather than general care.
For example:

*Q. Mrs Enid Andrews, aged 43 years, is married and has a 12-year-old
daughter. She is admitted at 02.00 hours with acute intestinal obstruction,
thought to be due to adhesions following a previous appendicectomy.*
*(a) Describe the nursing measures likely to be taken until Mrs Andrews
goes to the operating theatre,* 60%
*(b) Describe the nursing care Mrs Andrews will require during the first six
hours after the operation.* 40%

Final R.G.N. Paper, English and Welsh National Board, July 1984

(*a*) requires only information about your care in the period between her
admission to the ward and her arrival in the operating theatre.

(*b*) requires only information about your care in the immediate postoperative period.

The weighting (60 per cent (*a*), 40 per cent (*b*)) means that the examiner expects more detail in (*a*) and you should take this into account in your answers.

Q. Mr Paul Cox, a 37-year-old executive, is admitted to hospital, while on a business trip, with a perforated duodenal ulcer. He is married, smokes and leads a demanding social life.
(a) Give an account of Mr Cox's specific preoperative care following his admission to the ward. 60%
(b) What postoperative advice will facilitate Mr Cox's initial recovery and eventual convalescence? 40%

Final R.G.N. paper, English and Welsh National Board, May 1984

(*a*) requires only the specific care needed by a gentleman with an acute abdominal problem during the period after his admission up to his transfer to theatre for emergency surgery.

(*b*) requires information about two aspects of his postoperative care; firstly, relating to how you can best advise him in the initial period following surgery and, secondly, how you can advise him in relation to his convalescence. In the second part you should show you are aware of the stress factors associated with his condition and explain the measures he can take to help reduce them.

7.2. Preoperative care

Initial nursing assessment

The information obtained from this is needed in order to plan the care and identify actual and potential problem areas for the patient.

If you are asked a question about assessing a patient prior to surgery then the question will normally tell you the age, sex and reason for admission. You need to show the examiner that you would consider the following areas when preparing your plan of care:
1. Family situation, e.g. next of kin; whether married or separated; living with parent; living alone or with others; how many dependants – are they living at home?
2. Social situation, e.g. occupation if employed; what effect does illness have on job? If unemployed, will there be difficulties with D.H.S.S. benefits? Culture and language.
3. Psychological state, e.g. is patient anxious and why? Has he been in hospital before? Are there any psychiatric problems?

4. Physical state, e.g. general health, including fitness, smoking, alcohol, medication; specific health relating to reason for admission; baseline physical assessment, e.g. temperature, pulse, blood pressure, respirations, urine test, weight; other significant information, e.g. diet, continence. You should also consider specific topics you may need to ask about relevant to the question. If, for instance, the question says the patient is diabetic and being admitted for repair of a hernia, you would still have to include questions relating to his diabetes in your assessment, although it is not the main reason for admission.

The admission procedure

If asked about the admission procedure you would need to include information about the nursing assessment in general terms and emphasize:
1. the friendly, caring approach, e.g. offer tea to the patient and relatives to help them relax; take your time to complete the relevant documentation with the patient
2. orientation to the ward/facilities
3. introduction to staff, other patients
4. explanation of ward routine
5. reasons for recording of observations.

If the admission is of an acutely ill patient who is going to theatre imminently, then you must show the examiner you are aware of the significant relevant factors associated with his condition.

Concentrate on important information: next of kin; informing relatives; reassurance/explanation; frequent observations; physical preparation for theatre as appropriate to his condition; specific care relating to his condition.

Preoperative preparation

Physical preparation
Pain relief (where appropriate)
Dietary build-up or restrictions
Exercises – deep breathing and/or other muscles
Bowel preparation (where relevant)
Skin preparation: do not just write down 'operation site is shaved'; show the examiner you know where the area is, e.g. for Mr Smith, a 60-year-old, prior to the repair of bilateral inguinal hernias, the lower abdominal and pubic area would be shaved.

Aspects of general nursing care appropriate to the patient's condition, e.g. mouth care in a dehydrated patient; pressure area care in an immobile patient.

Psychological preparation
Orientation to ward

Explanation of procedures

Involve relatives where appropriate

Explanation/discussion of patient's understanding of the planned operation

Reassurance of patient's anxieties, e.g. postoperative pain, medication, tubes

Mention of appropriate referrals, e.g. to the physiotherapist, dietitian, and medical social worker should be included in either physical or psychological preparation where necessary.

Investigations
Reference should be made only to relevant investigations.

1. Electrocardiogram for anyone who may have a cardiac problem or who is elderly.

2. X-rays must be written specifically, e.g. abdominal X-ray for a patient with acute abdominal obstruction; neck X-ray for a patient with thyroid goitre; chest X-ray for a patient with a lung lesion or routinely to detect lung problems prior to anaesthesia.

3. Blood tests should be stated clearly and not referred to in a general sense. Most patients will have a blood test for haemoglobin concentration and white cell count *but* grouping and cross-matching is *not* required for most smaller surgical procedures although urea and electrolyte levels are often measured routinely.

4. If there are significant specific investigations that are carried out, e.g. a cholecystogram for a patient with suspected gall stones, then this should be stated.

5. Do not spend too long writing in detail about medical tests and investigations. It will normally suffice to say, for example, for Mr Smith, a 60-year-old gentleman, prior to repair of an inguinal hernia: an electrocardiogram and chest X-ray were carried out and a blood specimen tested for haemoglobin and white cell count to ensure Mr Smith was fit for surgery. The nurse ensured that the results and X-ray were sent to the theatre with Mr Smith.

Checklist prior to theatre

You will be familiar with the checklist used in your hospital and it should include the following checks on the patient:

1. His identity is correct.
2. The consent form has been signed.
3. Notes, X-rays and other test results are available.
4. The appropriate area of the body has been shaved/prepared.
5. Jewellery/prostheses have been removed.
6. The premedication has been given and the time recorded.
7. There has been no oral intake for the prescribed time.
8. Valuables have been locked away safely.
9. The patient has washed and is gowned appropriately.
10. The last time the patient voided urine is recorded.
11. The last measurements of pulse, blood pressure, temperature, respirations and weight are included on the relevant chart.

7.3. The recovery room

Most hospitals have recovery areas within the theatre complex where patients are nursed until regaining consciousness before transfer back to the ward. However, this is not always so and when answering a question relating to immediate postoperative care it is important to show the examiner that you are aware of the potential problems following anaesthesia.

In the recovery room the following nursing assessments would be made:

1. *Respiratory status*

Depth, rate and rhythm

Colour – peripheral and central

Early detection of airway obstruction due for example to secretions or relaxation of the tongue.

2. *Cardiovascular status*

Heart rate, rhythm, blood pressure

Early detection of hypotension, hypertension and arrhythmias.

3. *Neurological status*

Level of consciousness

Response to stimuli/command

Indications that the effect of the anaesthetic drugs and muscle relaxants have worn off, e.g. ability to move limbs voluntarily.

4. *Other aspects of management*

Urine output

Drainage from wound drains
Temperature control especially if patient is hypothermic
Recording of other monitoring data, e.g. central venous pressure
Correct oxygen administration
Care of oral airway
Care of intravenous infusions
Administration of prescribed analgesia
Control of nausea and vomiting
Psychological support for the patient.

7.4. Postoperative care

It is very important to read the question carefully when asked about postoperative care.

If the question says *plan care for the first six hours following surgery*, then that is what you must do. Write in detail about this period and do not include what happens the next day and so on, as you will not get any marks for information which was not requested.

If the question says *plan care for forty-eight hours following return to the ward from the recovery area* then your answer must concentrate on care during this period. You can assume that the patient is already conscious and plan care accordingly.

If the question says *using a problem-solving approach plan care following surgery until discharge* then you must identify problems in your answer. Also as the question covers the entire postoperative period you must not spend twenty-five minutes writing about the first six hours and ten minutes about the next ten days but balance your answer so as to produce an account of care for the whole period.

Initial phase

Some preparation should be made before the patient's arrival on the ward. This should include:
1. ensuring oxygen and suction equipment is available
2. positioning the bed in the ward so as to allow appropriate observation, e.g. near nurses' station if following major surgery
3. preparing the bed with appropriate sheets/pillows
4. having available specific other equipment required, e.g. IVI stand, catheter-bag stand, mouth-care pack, sphygmomanometer, etc.

The specific preparation required will depend on the type of surgery and the individual problems identified in the preoperative care plan. On arrival on the ward the nurse must:

1. ensure safe transfer of patient from theatre trolley to ward bed;

2. obtain an accurate report from recovery nurse relating to operation, anaesthesia and recovery room care;

3. check patient's identity;

4. check wound site;

5. ensure observation charts/Kardex/medical prescriptions are up to date.

The immediate care plan must consider problems as in the recovery room, and observations of vital signs should be made frequently, e.g. quarter- to half-hourly for two hours; hourly for four hours; four-hourly for forty-eight hours. More frequent observations are made following major surgery or if the patient develops cardiovascular or respiratory problems.

Important points to include in your plan of patient care for the initial postoperative phase are:

1. *Maintenance of airway*
Nurse semi-prone until conscious
Observe and record respiratory rate, depth and rhythm
Administer oxygen as prescribed
Sit up as condition improves.

2. *Observation and recording of vital signs*
Level of consciousness
Pulse/heart rate and rhythm
Colour of skin – peripherally and centrally
Temperature
Blood pressure.

3. *Observation and care of*
Intravenous infusion (if appropriate)
Wound site/dressing
Wound drains
Nasogastric tube (if appropriate)
Urinary output.

4. *Pain relief*
Give regular analgesia as prescribed, e.g. Omnopon 15 mg intramuscularly four-hourly is a good example of a typical postoperative régime.

These points should be emphasized and described in detail if the question relates only to care for the first few hours following surgery.

Other aspects should be included but the above should be recorded early in your answer to show the examiner that you appreciate the importance of them.

Total management

The content of an answer to a question on postoperative management is best considered by a worked example.

Q. Peter Stevens is a 46-year-old company executive who is married with two teenage children. He has undergone emergency surgery for a perforated appendix and has been transferred to the ward from the recovery area of the theatre.

Using a problem-solving approach, plan his care from the time of his transfer to the ward until his discharge home. 100%

When planning his care you need to take into account his age, occupation and family situation as well as the specific postoperative nursing care required. You can use any model of nursing with which you are familiar as a basis for your answer or produce the answer in an essay form as long as you use a problem-solving approach, identify actual and potential problems, and explain appropriate nursing action.

The following answer is not based on a specific model but contains the information which you would be expected to include in your answer.

Problems	Nursing Action
Potential difficulty with breathing due to anaesthesia or development of chest infection	1. Nurse semi-prone until conscious. 2. Sit up when condition permits. 3. Encourage deep breathing. 4. Encourage expectoration of secretions. 5. Record and observe respiratory rate, depth and rhythm half-hourly initially, then decrease observations as condition improves. 6. If chest infection develops give inhalations and prescribed antibiotics.
Pain	1. Give intramuscular analgesia, e.g. Omnopon, 15 mg regularly as prescribed. 2. After twenty-four to forty-eight

Problems	Nursing Action
	hours give prescribed oral analgesia, e.g. Paramol, two tablets six-hourly as required. 3. Evaluate effect of analgesia given. 4. Change his position to help reduce pain, 5. Encourage him to rest especially in first forty-eight hours.
Difficulty with hygiene	1. Wash face and hands when conscious. 2. Change theatre gown for pyjamas. 3. Give him a blanket bath on day 1 postoperatively. 4. Help with washing, as condition permits on subsequent days. 5. Give oral care while nil orally/restricted fluids. 6. Assess him for other areas of personal hygiene needs, e.g. hair, skin. 7. Encourage him to take responsibility for his own hygiene needs as soon as he is able.
Restricted oral intake	1. Initially give nil orally 2. When instructed by the surgeon give ice to suck and gradually increase fluids. 3. Aspirate and record nasogastric aspiration as instructed. 4. Give oral/nasal care and offer mouthwashes. 5. Encourage fluid intake and diet when peristalsis returns. 6. Maintain as prescribed intravenous fluid replacement. 7. Maintain an accurate fluid balance chart.
Immobility	1. Change position two-hourly while on bed rest. 2. Use appropriate aids, e.g. sheepskin.

Problems	Nursing Action
	3. Observe pressure areas two-hourly.
	4. Encourage movement and exercises.
	5. Sit out of bed on day one for short periods if possible.
	6. Encourage early ambulation with realistic goals.
Difficulty with elimination: Urinary retention	1. Ensure urinal is easily available.
	2. Ensure privacy and preserve dignity.
	3. Help to sit on edge of bed or commode if condition permits.
	4. Observe and monitor urinary output.
	5. Encourage to use toilet when able.
Constipation	1. Give aperients if prescribed.
	2. Encourage to use toilet when able.
	3. Ensure privacy.
Anxiety, about operation, family or work	1. Listen and talk to Mr Stevens; answer his questions honestly.
	2. Explain operation and postoperative care.
	3. Involve him in his care.
	4. Encourage family to visit.
	5. Refer to other agencies if necessary.
	6. Explain discharge/follow-up arrangements.
Potential problems: Wound infection	1. Observe wound for evidence of infection, e.g. inflammation.
	2. Record temperature four- to six-hourly.
	3. Care of wound drain.
	4. Remove or shorten wound drain as required.
	5. Always use aseptic technique.
	6. Send swabs for microscopy culture and sensitivity if infection suspected.
	7. Remove sutures on day five to seven

Problems	Nursing Action
	depending on state of wound/surgeon's instructions.
	8. Give antibiotics as prescribed.
Cardiovascular changes, e.g. shock/haemorrhage, deep vein thrombosis	1. Observe skin colour – peripheral and central.
	2. Monitor pulse and blood pressure frequently initially; reduce observations as condition permits.
	3. Encourage leg exercises to prevent deep vein thrombosis and/or fit thromboembolic stockings.
Nausea and vomiting	1. Give appropriate antiemetics as prescribed.
	2. Ensure bowl and tissues within his reach.

Preparation for discharge

This is an important part of postoperative care and should be an ongoing consideration throughout the postoperative period.

Points to consider when planning discharge are:

1. Involve the patient and family/friends at an early stage.
2. Which community agencies need to be involved? (See Chapter 4.)
3. Is there a need for convalescence?
4. Is he ready for discharge – physically and psychologically?
5. Is the home situation satisfactory?
6. Can he or the family manage any treatment, e.g. injections/colostomy care, that is required?
7. Do they know how to get supplies?
8. Does the patient understand about his medication?
9. What restrictions must the patient make to his lifestyle?
10. Have outpatient/follow-up appointments been made?
11. Does transport need to be organized for the appointments or discharge?

7.5. Asepsis

Aseptic techniques are vital during surgery and when carrying out wound dressing procedures.

The aim of an aseptic technique is to prevent infection.

Key facts of the principles of asepsis

1. Limit airborne contamination.
2. Use a non-touch technique.
3. Wash hands appropriately to remove contaminants.
4. Prepare and dispose of equipment correctly.
5. Limit exposure time of wound to a minimum.
   The above are achieved by:
   1. preparing the patient mentally and physically
   2. preparing the area surrounding the patient
   3. preparing the equipment
   4. cleaning hands at appropriate times and in the correct way
   5. carrying out non-touch technique without causing any contamination
   6. responding to the patient's needs appropriately
   7. disposing correctly of equipment used/contaminated dressings
   8. cleaning dressing trolley correctly
   9. carrying out procedure quickly and efficiently
   10. reporting relevant observations about condition of the wound
   11. taking wound swabs where appropriate.

8. Care of patients with neurological problems

8.1. Introduction

Some key facts relating to the anatomy and physiology of the nervous
system are included in this chapter but these alone do not cover the depth
of knowledge which the student should possess. An appropriate source
of reference would be *Penguin Masterstudies: Biology*, Chapter 7. A short
section on terminology associated with care of patients with neurological
problems is also included.

This chapter covers the key points of care associated with the major
neurological problems with which the student must be familiar. Most
examination papers contain a question relating to one of the topics
covered in this chapter. Nursing care of an unconscious patient is also
included here as it is often linked in examination papers to care of patients
following head injuries or cerebral bleeding.

8.2. Key facts relating to anatomy and physiology

The brain and spinal cord are covered by three layers of *meninges* – dura,
arachnoid and pia.

The cerebrum is divided into left and right cerebral hemispheres, each
of which have a frontal, parietal, temporal and occipital lobe.

The vital centres for the control of respiration, heart rate and blood pressure are located in the *medulla*, as are the centres for the integration of the responses (reflexes) associated with swallowing, coughing and vomiting. The *hypothalamus* contains the centre for temperature regulation. The *cerebellum* is the centre for the co-ordination and control of muscles and balance.

The *internal capsule* is the area where the bundles of nerve fibres exit from the cerebral hemispheres to enter the brainstem prior to 'crossing over' (decussation).

The *cerebrospinal fluid* is formed in the *choroid plexuses* and is absorbed by the *arachnoid villi*. Its normal pressure when lying down is approximately 130 mm H_2O. It is normally a clear solution which forms a protective covering for the brain and acts as a cushion in the event of injury as well as providing uniform pressure around the brain at all times.

The examiners would expect you to know the names of the cranial nerves and their major effects as well as being able to draw a simple reflex arc and identify the major pathways associated with touch, pain and temperature.

Summary of key effects of the sympathetic and parasympathetic nervous system

	Sympathetic	Parasympathetic
Pupil	Dilates	Constricts
Bronchi	Dilates	Constricts
Cerebral blood vessels	Constricts	Dilates
Coronary blood vessels	Dilates	Constricts
Skin blood vessels	Constricts	No fibres present
Heart rate	Increases	Decreases
Digestive tract	↓persistalsis	↑peristalsis
Urinary sphincter	Closes	Opens
Urinary bladder (smooth muscle)	Relaxes	Contracts
Sweat glands	Stimulates secretion	No fibres present

8.3. Terminology

Aphonia: absence or loss of voice
Anosmia: absence of smell
Babinski reflex: a pathological extension – plantar reflex
Dysarthria: disorder of articulation
Dysphagia: difficulty in swallowing

Dysphasia: disorder of language. There are two main types:
1. receptive – the impairment of comprehension of language
2. expressive – disorder of the expression of language

Encephalitis: infection of the brain tissue

Hemianopia: blindness in half of the visual field

Hemiplegia: paralysis of one side of the body

Hydrocephalus: an excessive accumulation of cerebrospinal fluid due to obstruction of the circulation or inadequate absorption of the cerebrospinal fluid

Ipsilateral: same-sided

Otorrhea: discharge (e.g. leak of cerebrospinal fluid) from the ears

Paraesthesiae: 'pins and needles'

Paresis: weakness

Plegia: paralysis

Rhinorrhea: discharge (e.g. leak of cerebrospinal fluid) from the nose.

8.4. Neurological assessment of patients

It is not sufficient to write down 'neurological observations were carried out' or 'pupil reaction was tested', when answering questions. The examiner expects you to understand why you are carrying out the observations and also the significance of what you observe on assessment.

If you are familiar with the neurological assessment chart used in your hospital, then this would serve as a good basis for checking the points to be considered. If not, the chart reproduced opposite is widely used and an internationally accepted one:

The assessment is considered in this chapter in the following categories:
1. Conscious level
2. Pupil reaction
3. Limb movement
4. Vital signs

1. *Conscious level.* Is the patient alert, opening his eyes when you approach, or does he require stimulation to open them? If so, is it as a result of speech or as a response to pain? Is there no response at all?

When he responds to speech, is he orientated in time, place and person, or is he confused or demonstrating a speech defect, e.g. receptive or expressive dysphasia? Is he only uttering incomprehensible sounds or making no response at all?

Does he obey commands, e.g. 'squeeze my hand', or does he only

INSTITUTE OF NEUROLOGICAL SCIENCES, GLASGOW
OBSERVATION CHART

| NAME | | | DATE |
| RECORD No. | | | TIME |

C O M A	Eyes open	Spontaneously		Eyes closed by swelling = C
		To speech		
		To pain		
		None		
S C A L E	Best verbal response	Orientated		Endotracheal tube or tracheostomy = T
		Confused		
		Inappropriate Words		
		Incomprehensible Sounds		
		None		
	Best motor response	Obey commands		Usually record the best arm response
		Localise pain		
		Flexion to pain		
		Extension to pain		
		None		

Pupil scale (m.m.)
• 1
● 2
● 3
● 4
● 5
● 6
● 7
● 8

Blood pressure and Pulse rate
240
230
220
210
200
190
180
170
160
150
140
130
120
110
100
90
80
70
60
50
40
30
Respiration 20
10

Temperature °C
40
39
38
37
36
35
34
33
32
31
30

PUPILS	right	Size		+ reacts
		Reaction		− no reaction
	left	Size		c. eye closed
		Reaction		

LIMB MOVEMENT	ARMS	Normal power		Record right (R) and left (L) separately if there is a difference between the two sides
		Mild weakness		
		Severe weakness		
		Spastic flexion		
		Extension		
		No response		
	LEGS	Normal power		
		Mild weakness		
		Severe weakness		
		Extension		
		No response		

respond to painful stimuli? If so, is it a localizing response or an example of a flexion and extension response? Is there no response at all?

2. *Pupil reaction.* What size are his pupils? Are they regular in shape and are they equal? Do they respond equally to light and is that response brisk or sluggish?

3. *Limb movement.* Are the limbs being moved spontaneously with normal power? Is there any evidence of mild or severe weakness? Is spastic flexion evident in the arms or extension evident in the arms or legs? Is there any 'twitching'? Is there no response at all?

4. *Vital signs.* This includes recording of temperature, pulse, respirations and blood pressure for all patients.

You would not be expected in the R.G.N. examination to know what the specific tests for the individual cranial nerve functions are.

The most important reason for carrying out frequent neurological assessment is to identify any changes in the patient's condition. Changes which may be associated with an increase in intracranial pressure are:

1. ↑temperature as a result of damage to the heat-regulating centre in the hypothalamus

2. ↓pulse as a result of damage to the cardio-inhibitory centre

3. ↑blood pressure due to the effects of cerebral hypoxia stimulating the vasomotor centre

4. ↓respiratory rate due to damage to the respiratory centre

5. a deterioration in the level of consciousness as assessed in section (1) above

6. an increasing dilatation of the pupils

7. a deterioration in limb movement, e.g. evidence of a greater weakness than previously or a change from the limbs being held in a normal position to an extension position

8. headache, presence of; increasing severity; frequency or duration.

Other associated points to consider when making a neurological assessment are:

1. Has the patient been taking drugs which could cause a change in pupil reaction? – e.g. narcotics cause constriction.

2. Are there other general signs which could indicate cerebral changes? – e.g. ↑restlessness may be due to cerebral irritation.

3. Is there neck stiffness which may be indicative of meningitis or a subarachnoid haemorrhage?

8.5. Care of the unconscious patient

When caring for an unconscious patient, there are two main areas to take into consideration. The first is the care required which is specific to the reasons for the patient's unconsciousness. If he is unconscious, for example, because of diabetic ketoacidosis then frequent assessment of blood sugar levels and administration of appropriate fluids and insulin are important factors. The second is the care which the nurse must give in order that the patient's normal daily needs can be satisfied. You may wish to use one of the nursing models as a basis for planning this care (see Chapter 2).

Always remember that the last sense that a patient loses when he is unconscious and the first that returns as he is regaining consciousness is hearing. It is very important always to assume that the patient can hear you and to talk to him about the care you are giving and keep him informed of day-to-day occurrences, e.g. weather conditions and world events.

The most important aspect of care relating to an unconscious patient must always be the establishment and maintenance of the airway and this should always be included in an examination answer at an early stage to indicate to the examiner that you appreciate the importance of this aspect of care.

Key aspects of nursing management

Establishment and maintenance of airway by:

1. Placing patient in a semi-prone position to prevent tongue obstructing airway and to promote drainage of secretions.

2. Insertion of oral airway or endotracheal tube if required to prevent airway obstruction and facilitate easier removal of secretions.

3. Removal of secretions from upper respiratory tract by helping the patient cough, if cough reflex is present. If cough reflex is absent use appropriate suction technique. Secretions removed from the lower respiratory tract via an endotracheal or tracheostomy tube *must* be removed using a *sterile* suction technique.

4. Promotion of ventilation to both lungs by two-hourly turning from side to side or a semi-prone position. Use of chest physiotherapy to assist coughing and promote loosening of secretions.

5. Regular observation of respiratory rate, depth, rhythm, and assessment of air entry to the chest so as to detect signs of deterioration or evidence of complications at an early stage, e.g. bronchopneumonia, respiratory muscle weakness.

6. Administration of oxygen as prescribed and care to ensure it is humidified to prevent drying of secretions and mucous membranes.

Assessment of neurological state and vital signs
As in section 8.4 (pages 118–20)
N.B. The frequency with which these observations would be carried out would depend on the condition of the patient but should never be less frequent than two-hourly, e.g. a patient receiving care immediately following a head injury should have the observations carried out quarter-hourly during the initial period. It is important to state what you are looking for when making these observations.

Maintenance of patient's daily needs
1. Mobility:
(a) Correct limb positioning and support of limbs.
(b) Passive limb exercises to all limbs at least four times daily.
2. Hygiene:
(a) Give bed bath at least daily, supplemented with other washes where appropriate, e.g. if patient is perspiring excessively.
(b) Carry out oral care two- to four-hourly as required, changing the airway, if *in situ*, frequently.
(c) Protect the eyes from corneal ulceration and drying by irrigation at least four-hourly with, for example, sterile saline solution. Use a pad if necessary and if eyes are held open close them using, for instance, a small piece of paraffin gauze.
(d) Carry out appropriate care to ears and nose and observe for evidence of leakage of cerebrospinal fluid if a basal skull fracture is suspected.
3. Drinking:
(a) DO NOT give oral fluids unless via a nasogastric tube into the stomach.
(b) Give intravenous fluids and/or nasogastric feeds as prescribed.
4. Elimination:
(a) Maintain an accurate fluid balance chart.
(b) Carry out catheter care if catheter *in situ*.
(c) Observe for retention or incontinence of urine and act appropriately.
(d) Ensure bowels are opened regularly. Give aperients when prescribed.
5. Communication:
(a) Talk to the patient, always explaining what you are doing.
(b) Establish communication by actions such as hand squeezing if patient is able to do this.

(c) Assess patient's response to speech, touch and presence of friends or relatives.

Prevention of complications
1. Deep vein thrombosis: exercise limbs, observe limbs for redness or swelling; use correctly fitting antiembolic stockings.
2. Pressure sores: turn two-hourly, inspect pressure areas for blanching, redness and signs of breakdown, use aids, e.g. a sheepskin; bedcradle to reduce pressure of bedclothes on toes.
3. Dehydration: maintain accurate fluid balance chart, observe skin turgor, observe urine for concentration.
4. Joint contraction and muscle wasting: ensure correct positioning of limbs; two-hourly passive exercises for all limbs; use of appropriate aids, e.g. footboard to prevent footdrop.

Relatives
Care, support and explanation of nursing actions to relatives is also of major importance when caring for an unconscious patient. This includes encouraging their participation in the patient's care if they wish, e.g. helping wash him, bringing tape recordings in for him to listen to, talking to him.

Other aspects of care
This includes administration of prescribed medication, e.g. antibiotics, anticonvulsants. Narcotics and sedatives are *not* normally prescribed because of their effect on the level of the patient's responsiveness making an accurate assessment of the patient's neurological state difficult. Care relating to investigative procedures, e.g. lumbar puncture, could also be included.

8.6. Specific care relating to major causes of neurological disturbances

Epilepsy

Key facts
1. Most epilepsy is idiopathic – no known cause.
2. Major conditions it can be associated with include cerebral trauma, infection, cerebral tumours, metabolic disorders and poisoning.
3. There are four main types of epilepsy:

(a) *Grand mal.* These are major seizures involving the entire brain and characterized by distinct phases.

The *aura* is a sensory experience the patient has prior to the seizure. It can involve any of the senses and may warn the patient sufficiently to enable him to protect himself. The aura does not always occur prior to a grand mal seizure.

The *tonic* phase is when the patient loses consciousness, cries out, arms are flexed, legs extended and the jaw becomes tightly closed. Respiration ceases and the patient may be incontinent.

The *clonic* phase follows and this is when breathing returns in a noisy, stertorous manner, the tongue may be bitten and profuse sweating may occur. The clonic and tonic phase are also known as the *ictus*.

The *postictal* (recovery) phase is when the patient appears drowsy and confused and needs to sleep. He may complain of a headache or muscle soreness.

(b) *Petit mal.* This is not preceded by an aura and the patient only loses consciousness transiently. There may be muscle twitching, loss of muscle control and the patient may stare vacantly while seeming confused. The entire attack may last only for approximately thirty seconds and recovery can be so rapid that the patient may not even be aware of the seizure.

(c) *Temporal lobe* (*psychomotor*). These can be associated with other physical and psychological disorders as well as paranormal phenomena, e.g. a *déjà vu* experience. They are characterized by purposeless, repetitive movements which the patient may be unaware of and may also involve a transient speech defect and emotional changes. The patient may be confused afterwards and have no recollection of the attack.

(d) *Jacksonian.* These are focal seizures that arise in the motor cortex. They may only involve one part of a limb, e.g. a hand, or may perhaps start at the neck and spread to include the arm and hand on the affected side.

4. *Status epilepticus* is a state of continuous grand mal fitting without a postictal phase.

5. Treatment is normally based on drug therapy and commonly used drugs include phenobarbitone, carbamazepine, Epilim and phenytoin.

You are most likely to be asked about patient care in relation to grand mal epileptic seizures and the following points relate to this, although the principles are applicable to any patient with seizures.

Key aspects of nursing management

During the attack

1. Prevent injury.

(a) Help patient to lie on the floor if not lying down and place in semi-prone position if possible to facilitate drainage of secretions and maintenance of airway.

(b) Loosen restrictive clothing.

(c) Remove surrounding objects, e.g. chair, locker, bed, from the immediate vicinity.

(d) Use pillows to prevent patient injuring himself on surrounding objects that cannot be removed, e.g. cotsides, bedhead.

(e) DO NOT force objects between clenched teeth.

(f) Remain with the patient.

2. Observe patient's behaviour

(a) Identify any precipitating factors, e.g. television programme.

(b) Was an aura present?

(c) Note the time and duration of the seizure.

(d) Note where it began anatomically and which parts of the body were involved.

(e) How long, if at all, was the patient unconscious?

(f) Did incontinence occur?

(g) Note the respiratory rate and pattern.

(h) Note deviation of the eyes and pupil changes.

(i) Were there any residual symptoms after the attack, e.g. weakness?

(j) How confused was the patient afterwards and could he remember the seizure occurring?

3. Preserve patient's dignity by screening area from observers

Following the seizure

1. Help patient into bed to rest.

2. Change soiled clothing.

3. Observe during rest for any further seizures.

4. When awake reorientate to surroundings.

5. Write an accurate record of events in the nursing Kardex.

Long-term care

1. Educate patient about the actions and toxic effects of the prescribed medication.

2. Stress importance of taking medication regularly.

3. Encourage patient to wear an identity bracelet.

4. Teach family and friends to care for the patient during seizures.
5. Give advice about driving licence.
6. Inform patient about British Epilepsy Association.
7. Warn parents of dangers of overprotecting children.
8. Give advice about avoiding boxing, swimming, climbing and factors which may precipitate attacks, e.g. stroboscopic lighting.
9. Discuss attitudes and understanding with patient and family.
10. Encourage parents to inform school.
11. Counselling about career limitations.

Head injury

Key facts
Damage to brain tissue may occur as a result of a skull fracture or acceleration or deceleration injuries.
1. *Skull fractures.* These can be simple, depressed or comminuted.

Depressed fractures always require treatment because of the increase in intracranial pressure resulting from the haematoma associated with the fracture.

Basal skull fractures can cause haemorrhage from ears, nose and pharynx. Leaking cerebrospinal fluid via the ears or nose may also be associated with such fractures.

Elevation of the fracture and removal of foreign bodies would be carried out in a specialist neurosurgical unit.

Fractures are not always associated with brain injury.
2. *Brain injury.* A *contrecoup* injury is one in which the impact is at the front but the brain tissue damaged is at the rear and it is caused by the brain 'bouncing' off the wall of the skull.

Concussion is jarring of the brain.

Contusion is bruising of the brain.

Amnesia and epilepsy may be associated with or follow brain injury. Serious neurological deficits can result from damage to brain tissue.
3. *Haematoma formation.* 3 types of haematoma may be associated with head injuries:
(a) Extra-dural: this is bleeding into the space between the skull and the dura and most often occurs in the temporal region due to rupture of the middle meningeal artery. It may be due to venous bleeding in a small number of patients. There is a lucid period between the time of the injury and the onset of the deterioration. This is because the dura and skull are strongly adherent thus confining the blood to a local area. However, once the local pressure is sufficient to cause neurological changes action must

be taken rapidly because the intracranial pressure will continue to rise due to the rapid accumulation of blood from the bleeding artery.

(b) Sub-dural: this is bleeding into the space between the arachnoid and the dura. It is usually venous in origin. It can be acute, subacute or chronic depending on the size of the vessel and the extent of bleeding. Because the dura and the arachnoid are easily separated the blood can spread freely over an entire hemisphere before causing generalized pressure symptoms.

(c) Intracerebral: this is much less common and is normally associated with the elderly. Scattered haemorrhages normally occur within the brain tissue itself.

Key aspects of nursing management

Patients who have sustained minor head injuries with little or no loss of consciousness will still be admitted to the ward for observation for twenty-four to forty-eight hours in case of complications developing. The nursing management in these cases is directed towards an early detection of problems by regularly assessing neurological function and vital signs. The nurse must be able to explain clearly to the patient the need for the frequent observations and why they are carried out. The nurse should also emphasize to the patient the importance of rest during this period and the necessity of remaining in bed, initially lying flat.

Questions in R.G.N. examinations are more usually about patients who are either 'drowsy and confused' or 'unconscious'. The management of these patients is obviously difficult in many aspects but you would definitely need to include details from 8.4. (neurological assessment) and 8.5. (unconscious patient) in your answer. For example, the following points should be considered.

Care relating to:

1. Maintenance of airway
2. assessment of conscious level, neurological function and vital signs
3. observation for complications, e.g. shock, cerebrospinal fluid leak
4. activities of daily living
5. participation in medical treatment, e.g. administration of steroids (dexamethasone), diuretics (mannitol), and restricted fluids to reduce cerebral oedema
6. support for family.

If the question asks for information relating to the observations you would make and their significance then you should confine your answer to what is asked but remember to include observations relating, for example, to urine output, skin condition, as well as those included in the neurological assessment.

Long-term effects

Serious neurological deficits can occur following serious head injuries and the rehabilitation may take many months if the patient has been unconscious for more than a few days. The family and patient need much support during this period. They need clear explanations as to the effects of the deficits and the patient needs to be encouraged to achieve those things that he is able to. He may benefit from joining organizations such as the Head Injuries Association.

There can also be major financial and social consequences following a serious head injury and appropriate support and referral for specialist advice and counselling should also be included in the plan of care.

Cerebrovascular accident (stroke)

Most cerebrovascular accidents are the result of an intracerebral haemorrhage, embolus or thrombosis. There is usually underlying cerebrovascular disease, e.g. atherosclerosis. Subarachnoid haemorrhage is considered (pp. 129–30) as specific aspects of the nursing care and treatment are different from those which apply to cerebrovascular accidents generally.

When answering questions relating to care of a patient following a cerebrovascular accident it is important to read the question carefully to ascertain whether the patient has suffered *a mild stroke* or has *a dense right hemiplegia* as the degree of disability will affect the content of the answer. It is also important to remember that:

1. A *right* cerebrovascular accident will cause *left*-sided symptoms and vice versa.
2. The main speech centre (Broca's area) is located in the left side of the brain; thus speech defects are most often associated with left cerebrovascular accidents.

Specific aspects of nursing management

Acute care

The first priority of nursing care in the acute phase must always be the maintenance of the airway. If the patient is unconscious then all care as in 8.5, pp. 121–3 should be given. If the patient is drowsy and confused much of this care is still appropriate as he will not be able to satisfy most of his daily needs himself.

In addition, it will be important to emphasize the care directed at maintaining safety, as a confused patient can easily fall out of bed, spill hot drinks or otherwise injure himself, especially when his confusion is combined with a physical disability, e.g. hemiplegia.

The acute phase lasts as long as the patient is unconscious or has to remain on bed rest. The correct positioning of limbs and regular passive exercises to paralysed limbs are vital during this phase in order to prevent contractures and other deformities which would create major problems in the rehabilitation phase.

The rehabilitation phase
This phase starts as soon as the patient regains consciousness or, if conscious initially, on the day that the stroke occurs.

An answer to a question about the rehabilitation of a patient with a hemiplegia, following a cerebrovascular accident, would need to include the following:
1. The importance of rehabilitation being a team effort involving medical staff, ward nursing staff, occupational therapists, physiotherapists, speech therapists, relatives, and later, community nurses.
2. A good assessment of the patient's deficits and abilities with realistic goals being set for the rehabilitation programme. Deficits which should be considered include:
communication problems, e.g. dysphasia
swallowing difficulty, e.g. dysphagia
difficulty with vision, e.g. diplopia
difficulty with movement, e.g. hemiplegia
and problems associated with micturition, defaecation, and a reduced ability to carry out other aspects of daily living as a result of the above problems (see specimen answer at the end of this chapter for details).

The rehabilitation phase does not end when the patient leaves hospital to return home but needs to be continued. Support for the patient and family can be given by the general practitioner, district nurse, occupational therapist, friends, neighbours and other relatives, the British Stroke Association, other agencies – statutory and voluntary as listed in Chapter 4 (pp. 73–5).

Education for the patient and family about residual deficits is important, e.g. accepting the disability; having realistic goals; allowing the patient to do what he can for himself; accepting emotional lability if present; appreciating that rehabilitation may take many months; the importance of discussing problems with professional staff, the hospital stroke unit or other voluntary agencies.

Subarachnoid haemorrhage

Subarachnoid haemorrhage is bleeding into the subarachnoid space from a ruptured aneurysm normally from an artery within the circle of Willis. It can be associated with congenital weakness of the artery wall but is also associated with hypertensive vascular disease. Unlike other cerebrovascular accidents, aneurysms have a tendency to rebleed.

Key aspects of nursing management

If the patient is unconscious then care is as described in 8.5 in addition to the specific points below.

If the patient is conscious then it is vital that everything is done to reduce a rise in intracranial pressure as this may cause a rebleed. This is achieved by the following:

1. The patient is kept on strict bed rest, lying flat with only one pillow.
2. All care is carried out for the patient to minimize his exertion, e.g. feeding him, washing him.
3. Medications to loosen stools, reduce the blood pressure, reduce cerebral oedema are given.
4. Antifibrinolytic drugs, e.g. Cyklokapron, may also be administered to delay the clot lysis and thus reduce the risk of a further bleed.
5. Measurements are taken to reduce stress and anxiety, e.g. a quiet environment, limited visiting, sedation if necessary, as an increase in stress can lead to increased arterial pressure.

When condition is stable, neurological observations can be carried out at a reduced frequency, i.e. two-hourly. Otherwise, all care is carried out as for any highly dependent patient. If the patient is likely to benefit from surgery, he will be transferred to a neurosurgical unit. If the bleed is to be treated conservatively, he will remain on bed rest until medical staff are satisfied that the chance of a rebleed has subsided and their rehabilitation programme will follow the same course as for any other cerebrovascular accident.

You will not be expected to be familiar with details relating to neurosurgical care for your R.G.N. examination but if you are taking an internally set examination and you have gained experience working in a neurosurgical unit, then you should revise this topic as it would be reasonable to expect you to know about it.

Lumbar puncture

A lumbar puncture is an investigation which you would be expected to know about as it is used diagnostically for a number of neurological problems. It is always carried out if a subarachnoid haemorrhage is suspected as in this procedure fluid from the subarachnoid space is withdrawn and evidence of bleeding would be found if a subarachnoid haemorrhage had occurred.

Nursing responsibilities
Prior to procedure: reassure and explain what will happen to the patient; prepare equipment and patient, e.g. empty bladder, position correctly, on left side, thighs and head flexed with a pillow under head and between legs.
During procedure: one nurse helps patient maintain position and explains the procedure to him; a second nurse assists the doctor including the collection of the specimens of cerebrospinal fluid.
Following procedure: help the patient to assume a comfortable lying-down position in bed. He is normally encouraged to rest for between six and twenty-four hours following lumbar puncture. This avoids the problem of post-lumbar puncture headache. The nurse should also carry out neurological observations as directed by the doctor and ensure the specimens of cerebrospinal fluid are sent quickly to the laboratory and all associated equipment is disposed of correctly. It is normal to apply a small waterproof dressing to the puncture site.

8.7. Other nervous system disorders

Multiple sclerosis

Key facts
1. A chronic progressive disease of the central nervous system
2. Characterized by demyelination of the white matter in the brain and spinal cord
3. Normally affects young adults aged 15 to 45 years
4. Occurs mainly in cold, damp (temperate) climates
5. May be associated with an autoimmune response
6. Normally characterized by relapses and remissions
7. Problems that patient complains of are associated with the sites affected, e.g. nystagmus, diplopia and blurred vision if cranial nerves II, III, IV or VI are affected
8. Motor weakness leading to spastic paralysis if the spinal cord is affected.

Key aspects of nursing management
1. Try to keep the patient as active and independent as possible.

2. Only assist the patient with tasks he really cannot perform.
3. The patient's ability will depend on the stage of the disease.
4. Prevent complications associated with bed rest.
5. Active muscle exercises should be encouraged and these supplemented with passive movements where necessary.
6. Good positioning to promote comfort and help prevent contractures.
7. Help to maintain safety – relate, for example, to visual disturbances, sensory loss and transfer from bed to chair.
8. Educate patient on use of aids and self-help devices.
9. Help him to re-establish regular toilet pattern if sphincter control is impaired.
10. Help him with psychological adjustments relating for example to mood swings, marital/relationship problems, rejection, grief process.
11. Advise the patient about Multiple Sclerosis Society, outings, clubs, holidays.
12. Give information about financial benefits and appropriate adaptations at home, e.g. Possum, non-slip mats, wheelchair ramps, wide doors.

Meningitis

This is an infection of the meninges and can be bacterial or viral in origin. The commonest infecting organisms are *neisseria meningitidis* (*meningococcus*), *streptococcus pneumoniae* and *Haemophilis influenzae*. It normally occurs secondary to an upper respiratory tract, ear or sinus infection.

Symptoms of which the patient may complain include headache, neck stiffness, fever, photophobia.

Key aspects of nursing management

1. Isolate patient until causative organism is identified.
2. Reduce fever by good air circulation, tepid sponging and fan therapy as prescribed, light bedclothes, cool fluids to drink or ice to suck and regular recording of temperature to assess the effect of the above.
3. Reduce pain by giving prescribed analgesia, e.g. codeine, and assess effectiveness.
4. Try to ensure a comfortable position and try not to disturb or move the patient unless absolutely necessary.
5. Position patient in a darkened side room to reduce photophobia.
6. Prevent dehydration by ensuring adequate fluid intake and maintaining an accurate record of fluid input and output.
7. Administer medication, e.g. antibiotics, antiemetics as prescribed.

8. Assess neurological state regularly and report changes. Remember that testing pupil reaction will be distressing for the patient so this should only be done when absolutely necessary.
9. Help with daily needs in relation to hygiene, nutrition and elimination, bearing in mind that the patient may be lying flat on bed rest initially.
10. Explain to patient and relatives about the darkened side room, need for quiet, restriction of visitors and need for investigations, e.g. lumbar puncture. Explain about the treatment and care, listen to their anxieties, answer their questions when able and refer to medical staff where appropriate.

8.8. Specimen R.G.N. questions

Q.1. Mrs Jackson, a 46-year-old housewife, has been involved in a road traffic accident while out shopping. She has been admitted to the ward with a head injury and is conscious but drowsy.

Identify Mrs Jackson's likely problems and describe the care she will require over the next forty-eight hours. 100%

R.G.N. Final Examination, English and Welsh National Board, May 1985

Q.2. Mr John Davies, a 30-year-old married man, has been admitted to a medical ward. He is drowsy and complaining of severe headache. Investigations have confirmed a diagnosis of subarachnoid haemorrhage, which is to be treated conservatively.

Using a problem-solving approach, state how Mr Davies's care should be planned for the next three days. 100%

R.G.N. Final Examination, English and Welsh National Board, May 1984

8.9. Sample question and answer

Q. Mrs Phyllis Mead, a 64-year-old retired schoolmistress, is admitted to your ward, conscious but drowsy and with a left hemiplegia, following a cerebrovascular accident.
(a) Describe the observations that should be made during the first twelve hours, indicating the rationale for your actions. 40%

(*b*) *Describe the problems the hemiplegia may cause Mrs Mead and explain how the nurse can help her to minimize those effects during her stay in hospital.*   60%

(*a*) Observations must include:
1. respirations: rate, depth, rhythm, evidence of respiratory obstruction
2. pulse: rate, rhythm
3. blood pressure
4. temperature
5. neurological: level of consciousness, orientation time, place, person; response to stimuli and verbal commands; limb movement and power in plegic and normal limbs; pupil reaction: size equality.

The rationale for the above is to indicate changes associated with a rise in intracranial pressure and thus a deterioration in Mrs Mead's condition. Dilatation of only one pupil may indicate haematoma formation. Dilatation of both, ↑blood pressure, ↓pulse, ↓respirations and ↓conscious level, all could be indicative of raised intracranial pressure. Additional observations indicative of cerebral changes include: presence of headache, neck stiffness, visual changes, e.g. diplopia, photophobia, restlessness and vomiting. Other observations would be made on Mrs Mead, including:
1. generally, for evidence of any other injuries – she might have fallen when the stroke occurred
2. circulation and presence of pulses in affected side
3. skin condition for evidence of early breakdown
4. urine output for evidence of retention/incontinence
5. skin colour for evidence of circulatory/respiratory problems
6. skin textures for evidence of dehydration

(*b*) Hemiplegia may cause problems relating to:
movement in bed
ability to walk
feeding
washing/dressing
using the toilet
self-image.

You could answer this using a problem-solving approach or as an essay but the following details would need to be included.

When she is in bed ensure a two-hourly change of position, support of limbs, correct positioning, passive exercises to left arm and leg, and encourage Mrs Mead to exercise her right arm and leg. Teach her to exercise her left hand and arm by using her right hand. Cover the use of aids and slings to help with exercises. Teach her to transfer to a chair initially with help, how to stand with help, to walk with a frame or tripod. She would need help with feeding, especially if she has facial weakness, and appropriate aids should be provided. Special adaptations should be made to clothes to enable her to dress herself and she could be taught to use aids, e.g. for doing up/undoing buttons.

She will require help to wash but encourage her to do as much for herself as possible and set small increased goals as she manages previous targets. She will need help to get to the toilet and also to use a commode: teach her to use her good side to support herself.

Throughout the answer, it would be important to stress the multidiscipline involvement in her care and the setting of realistic goals throughout her programme. You should relate your care to minimizing the effects of the disability and not assume she will be completely cured although you will be aiming at the maximum degree of recovery possible.

You should include a paragraph on the effect of the hemiplegia on her psychologically and how it will affect her self-image and motivation; cause feelings of anger, frustration and disappointment when she cannot achieve; and you should indicate how you would try to minimize these effects by positively reinforcing achievements, discussing and planning her care with her, and ensuring that she is always treated with dignity – allowed time to dress properly and put her make-up on if she wishes.

8.10. Multiple choice questions

Q.1. An upper motor neurone lesion normally results in:
(a) *a flaccid paralysis*
(b) *loss of sensation*
(c) *a spastic paralysis*
(d) *marked muscle wasting.*

The correct answer is (c) because an increase in spastic tone occurs especially in the flexor muscles of the upper limb and extensor muscles of the lower limb. (a) is associated with a loss of tone and is indicative of a lower motor neurone lesion. (d) is also associated with a lower motor neurone and (b) is an effect caused by damage to sensory pathways.

Q.2. In addition to a decrease in respiratory rate and a deterioration in conscious level a rise in intracranial pressure is associated with which of the following?
(a) *hypertension, bradycardia, a sluggish dilated pupil*

(*b*) *hypotension, tachycardia, brisk dilated pupils*
(*c*) *hypertension, tachycardia, fixed constricted pupils*
(*d*) *hypotension, bradycardia, a brisk constricted pupil.*

The characteristic changes are hypertension and bradycardia. A sluggish dilated pupil would be indicative of an increased intracranial pressure, e.g. a haematoma. Thus the correct answer is (*a*).

Q.3. During which one of the following stages of a grand mal fit is incontinence like to occur?
(*a*) *aura*
(*b*) *recovery*
(*c*) *tonic*
(*d*) *clonic.*

The correct answer is (*c*).
N.B. Do not assume that the sequencing of events in the answer options reflects the sequence of events in the actual fit. Incontinence occurs during the second stage of the fit.

Q.4. Which of the following is correct when describing the sympathetic nervous system?
(*a*) *It is a three-neurone system.*
(*b*) *The chemical transmitter at the ganglion is acetylcholine.*
(*c*) *It is an afferent nerve system.*
(*d*) *It always complements the action of the parasympathetic system.*

It is only a two-neurone system via a ganglion and is a motor system consisting only of efferent fibres. It complements the action of the parasympathetic system in many areas but not always (see p. 117). The correct answer is (*b*) as acetylcholine is always the ganglion chemical transmitter.

9. Care of patients with respiratory problems

9.1. Introduction

This chapter is important because the general points considered apply to
many patients in hospital irrespective of their illness. Maintenance of the
airway is fundamentally important to life.

The relevant anatomy and physiology are not included in this chapter
but it is assumed that students would be familiar with the structure of the
respiratory system; the mechanics of breathing; the principles of blood
gas exchange; and the control of respiration. (See *Penguin Masterstudies:
Biology*, Chapter 3 for further details.) Some terminology is, however,
included as it is important to be aware of the meaning of words commonly
used in relation to patients with breathing difficulties.

Many examination questions, while not referring directly to a disease
process of the chest, expect you to be able to identify problems and plan
care relating to general respiratory difficulty or the prevention of chest
complications. For example, *Using a problem-solving approach describe
the nursing measures necessary to help Mrs Jones minimize the effects of
her dyspnoea and confusion.* Or *Plan Peter's care with specific reference to
the prevention of respiratory complications.*

9.2. Terminology/definitions and general points

Key words

Atalectasis: area of lung that is collapsed, airless and shrunken

Dead space: the part of a patient's tidal volume which does not take part in respiratory exchange

Emphysema: obstructive disease associated with destruction of the alveoli and dilatation of the air passages

Empyema: accumulation of purulent exudate in the pleural cavity

Haemoptysis: expiration of blood from the respiratory tract

Haemothorax: blood in the pleural cavity

Lobectomy: the surgical removal of one or more lobes of a lung

Minute volume: the amount of air breathed in or out in one minute

Pleurisy: inflammation of the surface of the pleura

Pneumonectomy: the removal of the entire lung

Pneumonia: an acute infection of the alveolar spaces of the lung

Pneumothorax: air in the pleural cavity

Tidal volume: volume of air breathed in or out in one breath

Vital capacity: greatest amount of air that can be breathed out after maximal inspiration

Oxygen therapy

Oxygen therapy should be prescribed by a doctor.

Safety precautions should always be taken, e.g. no smoking.

Oxygen should be humidified wherever possible to prevent drying of mucous membranes.

Patients with chronic respiratory disease should *not* be given high percentage O_2 as their respiratory drive is related to a decrease in blood oxygen levels and not to an increase in blood carbon dioxide levels as in healthy people without chronic chest disease. High percentage O_2 thus causes these patients to cease breathing if administration is prolonged.

General points to consider when assessing the following symptoms

1. *Cough*

Is it dry, wheezy, productive?

At what time of day does it occur?

Does anything stimulate it?

Is it associated with pain? If so, what type?

2. *Sputum*

What colour is it?
Is it thick and purulent, or thin and mucoid?
Is it offensive to smell?
Is it bloodstained, tinged pink or bright red and frothy?
Is its volume small or copious?
What is the risk of cross-infection?

3. *Dyspnoea*
When did it occur? Was the onset sudden?
Is it related to other problems, e.g. infection, cough?
Is it associated with exertion? If so, to what degree?
Is it related to an expiratory wheeze?
Is there associated cardiovascular disease?
Is orthopnoea present?
Is it related to anxiety?

4. *Chest pain*
Is it sharp and stabbing, or dull and aching?
Is it related to respiration?
Is it intermittent or continuous?
Where is the pain located?
What precipitates the pain?
Is it worse in a particular position, e.g. lying on left side only?

General points to be considered when caring for patients with respiratory difficulties

1. *Position in ward*: well ventilated; no draughts; easily observable; call bell within reach.
2. *Position in bed/chair*: sitting upright; well supported with pillows; orthopnoeic position.
3. *Administration of prescribed treatment and monitoring effects*: humidified oxygen (normally low percentage; respiratory stimulants, e.g. doxapram; bronchodilators, e.g. salbutamol, aminophylline.
4. *Assessment of vital signs*: respiratory rate, depth, rhythm, equality of chest movement; abnormal respiratory sounds, e.g. wheeze; temperature and pulse rate; degree, if any, of cyanosis; changes in conscious level (due to hypoxia), e.g. restlessness; confusion.
5. *Appropriate physiotherapy*: deep breathing; postural drainage; chest physiotherapy; use of expectorants if prescribed; regular change of position.
6. *Infection*: obtain sputum specimen and send to laboratory for microscopy, culture and sensitivity; ensure patient has tissues, sputum pot and bag available; correctly dispose of the above after use; administer

prescribed antibiotics; remove secretions by correct suction technique if necessary.

7. *Ensure adequate rest/prevent unnecessary exertion*: help with activities of daily living; ensure locker, urinal, commode within easy reach.

8. *Pain*: small, regular amounts of prescribed analgesia and monitor effect; comfortable position, support chest when coughing.

In addition, you should consider care relating to any patient confined to bed or with reduced mobility, e.g. prevention of pressure sores; promotion of good nutritional and fluid intake; maintenance of dignity; clear explanations of care and psychological support.

9.3. Specific care relating to causes of respiratory difficulty

The conditions included in this section are those with which students should be familiar and represent the topics most commonly asked about in examination questions.

Asthma

Key facts
1. An acute attack is associated with:
chest tightness
cough – dry initially→ productive
dyspnoea – especially on expiration
wheeze
mucosal oedema
cyanosis, sweating, rapid weak pulse
bronchospasm.
2. The hyper-reactivity of the bronchi is due to many factors including allergic, emotional, hereditary, associated disease processes or unknown factors.
3. Drug treatment includes bronchodilators, e.g. salbutamol, to cause muscle relaxation; corticosteroids, e.g. prednisolone, to reduce mucosal inflammation; preventive drugs, e.g. Intal, which reduce hyper-reactivity. (N.B. Intravenous aminophylline and hydrocortisone may be given for serious attacks.)

Key aspects of nursing management

1. If the question is related to a child, ensure the care is appropriate to his age and family situation.
2. Monitor condition for evidence of deterioration/improvement or development of complications, e.g. chest infection.
3. Use non-feather pillows, covered mattress, cotton blankets.
4. Position in a well-ventilated room, near windows, easily observable.
5. Administer medications, high percentage humidified oxygen; encourage fluid intake.
6. Encourage most comfortable position, e.g orthopnoeic.
7. Give psychological support, explanation, reassurance.
8. Give appropriate advice about prevention of attacks, e.g. importance of taking medication; avoiding known allergic materials; promotion of good mental and physical health.

Pulmonary tuberculosis

Nowadays most people suffering from tuberculosis are treated at home or in the community via chest clinics or health centres. It is possible that you might be asked to discuss this condition as part of a question in relation to health education and the following are examples of the types of issue you should consider including in your answer:
1. Historical perspective
2. Relationship to poor housing, institutional/hostel accommodation
3. Socio-economically deprived groups
4. Ethnic minorities
5. Poor health care and health education in those groups most at risk, e.g. due to inability to understand language or mistrust of doctors
6. Importance of B.C.G. vaccination, Heaf test, Mantoux test
7. Screening/chest clinics
8. Contact tracing

Key facts

1. The causative organism is *Mycobacterium tuberculosis*.
2. It is spread by droplet infection, e.g. by coughing, sneezing.
3. Onset is insidious and extensive disease can occur before patient notices symptoms.
4. Patient normally complains of fatigue, malaise, slight fever, night sweating, cough, weight loss, dyspnoea, sputum production and haemoptysis.

5. When admitted to hospital, patients are often anaemic and poorly nourished.
6. It is a notifiable disease: contacts are traced.
7. It is treated by simultaneous administration of two or more drugs, e.g. isoniazid; rifampicin; streptomycin; para-aminosalicylic acid.
8. Respiratory isolation should take place while patient is infectious.

Key aspects of nursing management
1. Care related to problems as above
2. Respiratory isolation technique, i.e. side room; encourage patient to cover mouth when he coughs; appropriate disposal of tissues/sputum
3. Early morning sputum specimens
4. Administration of medications and observation for side effects
5. Education of patient and family on importance of continuing to take medication after discharge and attending outpatient department or chest clinic as instructed.

Pneumonia

Key facts
1. This is inflammation of the lung normally due to infection
2. It is spread by droplet infection
3. The causative organism is most often *Streptococcus pneumoniae*
4. Patient complains of high fever, dyspnoea, rapid respiratory rate, chest pain, sweating, cough and sputum production, confusion
5. Specific investigations include chest X-ray, E.C.G., blood gas analysis, sputum specimen.

Key aspects of nursing management
1. Care related to the problems as above
2. Administration of prescribed medication, e.g. antibiotics, analgesia and monitoring of effects
3. Full basic nursing care as patient will be on bed rest initially
4. Remember to relate your care specifically to the patient in question, i.e. if he has chronic obstructive airways disease then only administer low percentage oxygen.

Pulmonary embolism

Key facts
1. Obstruction of one or more pulmonary arteries by a thrombus, e.g. originating from a deep vein in the leg
2. Symptoms dependent on the size of the thrombus
3. Problems include dyspnoea, pain, tachycardia, weakness, increased respiratory rate, sometimes haemoptysis
4. A small pulmonary embolism is treated with anticoagulant therapy
5. A large pulmonary embolism is a major emergency requiring resuscitative measures.

Key aspects of nursing management
1. Care related to problems as identified above
2. Management of anticoagulation therapy, e.g. heparin infusion; oral warfarin; and monitoring for side effects, such as bruising, bleeding, blood in urine
3. Management of pain
4. Monitoring of vital signs
5. Gradual mobilization; encourage physiotherapy.

Chronic bronchitis

This is discussed in the specimen answer on pp. 148–9.

9.4. Procedures

Underwater seal drainage

The following points should be included in the nursing management
1. Explain to the patient about the apparatus – why it is there, what it is doing.
2. Ensure patient is sitting up or lying with damaged lung uppermost.
3. Arrange pillows and tubing so that there are no dependent loops, kinks or pressure constraints to prevent drainage.
4. Secure apparatus by pinning tube to the sheet and securing the bottle safely on the floor or in an appropriate carrier below the bed.
5. Ensure all connections are secure and well taped and apparatus is connected correctly:

Underwater seal drainage

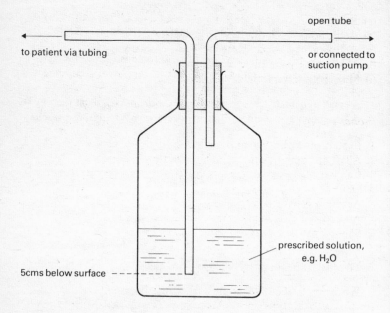

6. If bottle is not calibrated record volume of fluid which is instilled.
7. When 'milking' tube always milk towards the bottle.
8. Observe for oscillation, degree of bubbling and colour of any drainage.
9. If oscillation stops it could be due to a dependent loop, obstruction, or failure of the suction apparatus *but* it could also indicate that the lung is re-expanded.
10. *Never* raise the bottle above the level of the bed.
11. *Always* clamp the tube when changing the bottle.
12. Ensure two clamps are always available by the bed for use in emergency.
13. Encourage physiotherapy and early mobilization.
14. Administer prescribed analgesia and assess effect.
15. Teach junior nurses, other ward staff and visitors about the importance of not disturbing the apparatus.
16. When preparing for the removal of the tube:
(a) Explain procedure to patient.
(b) Administer prescribed analgesia.
(c) Prepare appropriate equipment maintaining asepsis.

(d) Ask patient to breathe in and out and then to breathe *in* deeply and hold his breath.

(e) Remove tube quickly. (N.B. Purse-string suture is normally *in situ*.)

(f) Apply firm dressing and seal adequately.

(g) Ask patient to *exhale* and then breathe normally.

(h) Dispose of equipment correctly and measure drainage.

(i) Make patient comfortable.

Bronchoscopy

1. Explain procedure to patient.
2. Allow nil orally six hours prior to procedure.
3. Carry out appropriate 'preoperative' safety checks (see Chapter 7 p. 108).
4. Accompany patient to endoscopy room.
5. Assist doctor in administration of local anaesthetic.
6. Support patient during procedure.
7. Position in semi-prone position ensuring airway patency initially.
8. Carry out observations to detect for evidence of complications, e.g. dyspnoea, cyanosis, bronchospasm, haemoptysis.
9. When cough reflex returns sips of fluid may be given.
10. Correctly label specimens obtained by doctor and dispatch to appropriate laboratory.

Tracheostomy care

Patients who have had severe respiratory difficulties or surgery involving the larynx may have a tracheostomy tube *in situ*.

Specific aspects to include in nursing management are:

1. Maintenance of airway by:

(a) appropriate position of patient to facilitate good lung expansion;

(b) safety of tracheostomy tube by correct inflation of balloon, use of tapes;

(c) removal of secretions by correct sterile technique;

(d) administration of humidified oxygen as prescribed.

2. Prevention of infection by:

(a) observing site for signs of infection;

(b) regular aseptic cleaning of site;

(c) use, for example, of 'keyhole' dressing;

(d) using sterile suction technique;

(e) sending regular sputum specimen to laboratory for microscopy, culture and sensitivity.

3. Ensure spare tracheostomy tubes of same and smaller size together with tracheal dilators are available by the bed for use in an emergency.

4. Give psychological support and explanations of care and treatment.

5. Teach patient to cover tracheostomy tube opening to speak or facilitate speech by using a speaking tube insert. Establish other means of the patient communicating his needs if this is not possible, e.g. writing, squeezing hand.

9.5. Thoracic surgery

The points considered in this section relate generally to patients undergoing thoracic surgery. It is important if answering a question on the subject to relate this also to the specific information given in the question. e.g. *Mr Smith has* carcinoma *of the* left *lung and is going to have a* pneumonectomy.

Key aspects of nursing management

Preoperative

1. Assist with pulmonary function tests/assessment.

2. Assess degree of breathing difficulty and plan nursing care accordingly, e.g. if chest infection present encourage fluids and administer prescribed antibiotics.

3. Stop patient smoking.

4. Discuss the surgery with patient and family, give support and refer family/patient for specialist counselling where necessary.

5. If patient is going to intensive therapy unit postoperatively arrange for a visit if possible or for patient to meet a nurse from the unit before surgery.

6. Teach patient about postoperative expectations, e.g. chest tubes and drainage; deep breathing exercises and chest physiotherapy; oxygen therapy; position in bed and turning; correct procedure for coughing.

7. Other preoperative preparation as discussed in Chapter 7 (pp. 106–8).

Postoperative

1. Maintain airway.

2. Position patient so as to avoid aspiration of fluids.

3. Give humidified oxygen as prescribed.

4. Apply sterile suction technique via endotracheal or tracheostomy tube if *in situ* or apply suction to oropharyngeal region as required.

5. Observe and record blood pressure, respiration and heart rate quarter- to half-hourly initially and reduce frequency as condition stabilizes.

6. Monitor chest drainage – volume, colour, amount.

7. Assist with coughing, deep breathing, leg and shoulder exercises.

8. Administer prescribed analgesia (small frequent doses are usually more effective than larger doses) and assess effectiveness as a patient in pain will not cough properly or breathe deeply and is thus more likely to develop complications.

9. Observe for evidence of complications, e.g. haemorrhage, respiratory failure, pulmonary oedema, pneumothorax and surgical emphysema.

10. Maintain and administer intravenous fluids or blood transfusion safely.

11. Administer prescribed medication, e.g. bronchodilators, antibiotics, and assess effect.

12. Maintain an accurate fluid balance chart of intake and output.

13. Mobilize as soon as possible, e.g. forty-eight hours postoperatively.

14. Encourage good walking posture.

15. Discuss patient's anxieties with him and provide support and health education, e.g. no smoking.

16. Ensure patient has adequate rest and a good diet, e.g. high protein, high carbohydrate, when he can tolerate it.

17. Other general postoperative care as discussed in Chapter 7 (pp. 109–10).

9.6. Specimen R.G.N. questions

Q.1. Mr John Atkinson, aged 65 years, who lives in a hostel for the homeless, has been admitted to hospital with a diagnosis of pulmonary tuberculosis and a history of haemoptysis. On admission he is lethargic and emaciated.

Identify Mr Atkinson's likely problems in the acute stage of his illness and indicate clearly the nursing action required to resolve each of these problems. 100%

R.G.N. Final Examination, English and Welsh National Board, January 1985

Q.2. Stuart Thorn, aged 19 years, is a member of the local athletics club. He is admitted via the accident and emergency department after having an underwater seal drain inserted for spontaneous pneumothorax.

(*a*) *How should the nurse explain to Stuart the cause of his condition and the purpose of the apparatus?*   35%

(*b*) *Describe the management of Stuart's underwater seal drain, including the removal of the tube after three days.*   65%

R.G.N. Final Examination, English and Welsh National Board, May 1985

9.7. Sample question and answer

Q. Mr Ian Reed, a 65-year-old retired bus driver, has been admitted to your ward with an acute exacerbation of chronic bronchitis. He is a heavy smoker and has been so most of his life.

(*a*) *Using a problem-solving approach discuss Mr Reed's nursing care during the first twenty-four hours following admission with particular reference to his respiratory problems.*   65%

(*b*) *Briefly describe the health education role of the nurse in the prevention of smoking.*   35%

(*a*) Note that the first part of the question carries a 65 per cent rating and therefore it is important to concentrate your answer on the specific aspects of the nursing care. The discussion should include the following problems and associated nursing actions.

1. *Dyspnoea.* Sit upright in bed, in a well-ventilated but not draughty position in the ward. Good support with pillows; easily observable position. Humidified low percentage O_2, e.g. 24 per cent as prescribed. Administration of appropriate drugs, e.g. salbutamol via nebulizer; aminophylline via intravenous infusion. Frequent observation of respiratory rate, depth, rhythm and peripheral and central colour.

2. *Cough/sputum.* Provide tissues, sputum pot, bag within easy reach, and change regularly. Administer expectorant as prescribed to help removal of secretions. Observe secretions for colour, texture and amount and send specimen to laboratory for microscopy, culture and sensitivity. Give moist inhalation. Regular chest physiotherapy, support when coughing.

3. *Anxiety.* Remain with Mr Reed initially. Orientate to immediate environment, and place locker and table within easy reach. Encourage relatives to remain with him but not to tire him. Explain clearly all procedures and the need for the oxygen mask and other treatment. Listen to him and discuss his anxieties with him as required.

4. *Pyrexia.* Monitor his temperature and pulse regularly and record

results. Administer prescribed antibiotics and observe for side effects. Provide cool pyjamas and cover only lightly with bedclothes. Have flannel available to wipe face frequently and change pyjamas and bed linen as required. Use fan therapy if necessary. Encourage fluid intake to help reduce effects of pyrexia and moisten secretions.

5. As a result of his respiratory problems he would have difficulty in looking after his own hygiene needs, e.g. oral care, washing. He would also, on account of being on bed rest during the first twenty-four hours, need help with his elimination needs and maintaining his mobility, e.g. regular change of position, limb physiotherapy. You could also include reference to maintaining his safety as he will be weak, distressed and possibly confused.

(b) The discussion should include the following points:

1. Emphasise that health education is directed at *everyone* not just smokers
2. Setting a role model example
3. Identification of problems caused as a result of smoking, e.g. respiratory tract infections; chronic bronchitis; peripheral vascular disease; coronary artery disease; carcinoma of the lung
4. Effect of smoking on non-smokers; antisocial effects; provision of literature; information on support groups, e.g. A.S.H.; involvement in programmes to help patients to stop smoking or referral to appropriate agencies.

You should relate the above information to your opportunities for counselling patients and relatives thus showing how you can contribute to this particular health education issue.

9.8. Multiple choice questions

Q.1. During the initial part of inspiration which one of the following statements is true?

(a) *intrapulmonary pressure decreases*
(b) *intra-abdominal pressure decreases*
(c) *intrathoracic pressure increases*
(d) *venous return to the heart decreases.*

The correct answer is (a) as otherwise air would be unable to enter the lungs. The other options are incorrect because during inspiration the intra-abdominal pressure increases as the diaphragm descends, the intrathoracic pressure decreases to allow the lungs to expand and these actions together increase venous return.

Q.2. A patient with chronic respiratory obstructive disease is ordered 26 per cent oxygen via a Ventimask. It is dangerous to exceed the amount ordered because:
(*a*) *the carbon dioxide levels in his blood are low*
(*b*) *oxygen tends to increase metabolism leading to dehydration*
(*c*) *his respiratory centre responds to lowered oxygen levels*
(*d*) *an increased respiratory sensitivity to carbon dioxide occurs.*

The correct answer is (*c*) as the main stimulus to breathing is hypoxia. The oxygen has no effect on respiratory sensitivity to carbon dioxide which is already impaired. It does not increase metabolism and the carbon dioxide levels would be high, not low, in this type of patient. Thus the other options are incorrect.

Q.3. Which one of the following characterizes an acute asthmatic attack?
(*a*) *pyrexia, chest pain, unproductive irritating cough*
(*b*) *bronchial dilation, decreased production of mucus, wheezing*
(*c*) *inspiratory difficulty, bronchial spasm, productive cough*
(*d*) *bronchial spasm, increased production of mucus, mucosal oedema.*

The correct answer is (*d*) as all factors included here are characteristic of an asthmatic attack. Asthma is not associated with bronchial dilation or characterized by inspiratory difficulty, chest pain or pyrexia although the latter may be present. Thus (*a*), (*b*) and (*c*) are incorrect.

10. Care of patients with cardiovascular and other circulatory problems

10.1. Introduction

An understanding of the heart and circulation is an important part of the
nurse's basic knowledge, as early detection of cardiac and circulatory
problems either in apparently healthy or ill patients is vital, and it is often
the nurse who is in a position to detect such.

The nurse needs to be aware of potential cardiac or vascular complications as a result of medical drug treatment or other aspects of patient
management, e.g. bed rest.

The nurse also has an important role in health education counselling
of patients and public in relation to promoting good health by making
them aware of the effects that diet, lifestyle and stress have on them. This
aspect of the role is of great importance when caring for patients who
have already developed arterial or vascular disease, as it is directed at
trying to lessen the risk of further progressive disease processes. This is a
topic on which students should ensure that they read current literature
prior to the examination as it may well be a subject chosen for the longer
question in the new internally set examination.

This chapter includes those topics most likely to be asked about in an
examination and considers the specific aspects of care relating to them
and other cardiac and vascular illnesses with which the student should be

familiar, as well as specific care relating to surgery of the arterial and vascular systems.

A number of commonly used drugs are mentioned in this chapter and students should ensure they are aware of their actions and side effects by reference to a suitable text, e.g. the current edition of the *British National Formulary* (published by the British Medical Association and the Pharmaceutical Press).

10.2. Key facts relating to anatomy and physiology

Anatomy

You should know the names and positions of the structures as shown in the diagram on p. 153 and also those involved in the conduction of the heart beat as shown in the diagram on p. 154.

The heart and circulation of blood

The outer covering of the heart is called the *pericardium* and consists of:
1. an outer fibrous pericardium
2. an inner serous pericardium with two smooth layers – *visceral* and *parietal*.

The middle layer of specialized cardiac muscle is called the *myocardium*. The inner endothelial lining is called the *endothelium*.

The *pulmonary circulation* carries *deoxygenated blood* from the *right ventricle* to the *lungs* and then returns the *oxygenated* blood to the *left atrium*.

The *systemic circulation* starts at the *aorta* and supplies all areas of the body with *oxygenated* blood and then returns *deoxygenated* blood to the heart finishing at the point of entry of the *inferior* and *superior venae cavae* into the *right atrium*.

The *portal circulation* drains the blood from the abdominal part of the digestive system via the *liver* to the *inferior vena cava*.

Blood vessels

Arteries and veins consist of three layers:
1. outer fibrous tissue – tunica adventitia
2. elastic and smooth muscle tissue – tunica media
3. inner endothelial layer – tunica intima

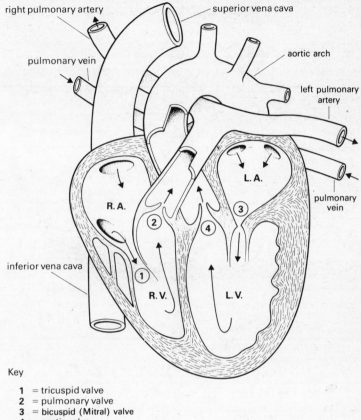

Key

1 = tricuspid valve
2 = pulmonary valve
3 = bicuspid (Mitral) valve
4 = aortic valve
R = right
L = left
V = ventricle
A = atrium
⟶ = direction of blood flow

Large arteries have a small amount of smooth muscle and a large amount of elastic tissue.

Arterioles have a small amount of elastic and a large amount of smooth muscle tissue.

Veins have a thinner tunica media with less muscle and elastic tissue.

Capillaries have only a single endothelial cell layer for their wall and no muscle, elastic or fibrous tissue.

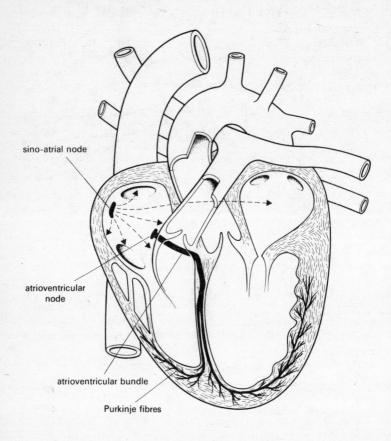

sino-atrial node

atrioventricular node

atrioventricular bundle

Purkinje fibres

Physiology

The sequence of events by which the heart pumps blood is known as the *cardiac cycle*. The ventricular contraction phase is known as *systole*. The ventricular relaxation phase is known as *diastole*.

Cardiac output = stroke volume × heart rate

Stroke volume = volume at the start _ volume at the end
        of systole   of systole

Arterial blood = cardiac output × total peripheral resistance.
    pressure

Electrical conduction in the heart can be represented by an electrocardiograph trace (E.C.G.).

Depolarization of the myocardial cells corresponds to the *contraction* phase while *repolarization* corresponds to the *relaxation* phase.

The electrocardiogram trace

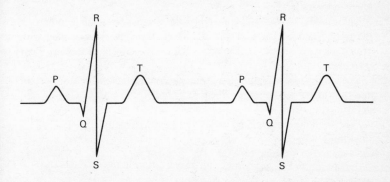

The P wave is produced by *atrial depolarization*. The QRS complex is produced by *ventricular depolarization*. The ST segment and T wave are produced by *ventricular repolarization*. The *atrial repolarization* effect is masked by the QRS complex.

The normal heart beats regularly in sinus rhythm.

Criteria for sinus rhythm
1. P–R interval is normal.
2. R–R interval remains constant.
3. P wave is followed by a QRS complex and followed by a T wave.
4. Rate is between 60 and 100 beats per minute.

N.B. You would not be expected to know about changes in E.C.G. traces as a result of abnormal pathology, but you should be able to identify and describe normal electrical conduction.

10.3. Health education

Arteriovascular disease, or arteriosclerosis, is an important cause of many cardiovascular and peripheral vascular problems. An important part of caring for patients suffering from these problems, in hospital and in the community, relates to identifying the 'at risk' factors in their individual cases and advising and helping them in the changes they may need to make in their lifestyles.

The nurse also has an important role to educate other members of the public and health professionals about the factors associated with arteriosclerosis and how people can reduce the effects of these in their own lives.

The nurse's role in health education is becoming increasingly important and thus examiners are more likely to include this aspect of nursing care in future questions.

'At risk' factors associated with arteriosclerosis include:
smoking
elevated serum cholesterol
elevated blood pressure
decreased levels of physical activity
dietary factors
personality type A (aggressive, competitive, impatient)
increased exposure to stress
family history.

The most serious illnesses associated with arteriosclerosis are those relating to coronary heart disease, e.g. angina, myocardial infarction.

All students should have nursed patients with these illnesses and would be expected not only to describe the practical care given, but to describe the health education advice given in relation to the factors identified. This should include consideration of the following:

1. Giving up smoking
2. Reducing stress in the working environment, e.g. assess the real need to work twenty hours per day or travel 300 miles per day in the car
3. Can changes in work pattern be made?
4. Are there specific stresses in the family/marriage/home situation which could be reduced?
5. What other stress factors are there in the person's life?
6. Decreasing intake of salt and cholesterol
7. Eating a greater proportion of polyunsaturated as compared to saturated fats in the fat component of the diet
8. Specific dietary advice with examples

 9. Advice to take regular *but not excessive* exercise
10. Reducing weight to optimum level if obese
11. Teaching the patient to relax.

Patients will need help if they are to undergo major changes in their lifestyle. The following can be involved in giving this support: close family; friends; members of the primary health care team; clinical nurse specialists, e.g. coronary care counsellors; support groups, e.g. post-myocardial infarct or post-amputee groups; relaxation groups; specialists, e.g. hypnotists, psychotherapists, to help them to give up smoking or identify ways to reduce stress.

The methods by which the public are made aware of the health education information regarding prevention of arteriosclerosis include broadcasts on radio and television; newspapers and magazines; government health warnings, e.g. on cigarette packets; Health Education Council publications; health education discussions at schools and colleges; lectures/ seminars by members of the primary health care team and other health care workers; campaigns by voluntary agencies, e.g. A.S.H.

10.4. Specific nursing care

Myocardial infarction

Key facts
Patients with actual or potential myocardial infarctions are normally admitted initially to a coronary care unit.

Problems they are likely to complain of include:
1. severe central chest pain often radiating to the neck and arm
2. nausea (and vomiting)
3. dyspnoea
4. sweating (with peripheral vasoconstriction)
5. faintness (especially if hypotensive).

Some but not necessarily all of the 'at risk' factors may be present – it will vary depending on the individual.

Key aspects of nursing management
Initially priorities of care are directed towards:
 1. assessment of vital signs, e.g. blood pressure, heart rate, respiration
 2. appropriate position in bed in relation to blood pressure
 3. administration of prescribed pain relief
 4. administration of prescribed humidified oxygen, e.g. 40 per cent via Ventimask

5. attaching to cardiac monitor. Observe; record rhythm
6. explanations of equipment and surroundings as appropriate
7. reassurance on anxieties as far as possible. Encourage patient to rest
8. obtaining nursing history from friend or relative as appropriate and including patient if able. Otherwise, wait until condition is stabilized
9. explaining to relative or friend about equipment, visiting, the need for patient to rest, availability of relatives' room if appropriate
10. assisting doctor with medical examination; insertion of intravenous cannula; recording of electrocardiogram.

After the initial assessment period the patient is likely to be on strict bed rest for at least forty-eight hours. During this period priorities of care include:

1. adequate pain relief
2. monitoring of vital signs regularly
3. observation of cardiac monitor and reporting of arrhythmias
4. promoting rest and quiet, ensuring appropriate bed position in ward
5. contrived administration of oxygen if necessary to relieve dyspnoea
6. controlling nausea if present
7. continued reassurance and explanations relating to equipment, procedures and other problems about which patient may be anxious
8. assistance with basic needs, e.g. hygiene, elimination
9. prevention of complications of bed rest, e.g. pressure sores, deep vein thrombosis; chest infection
10. provision of appropriate diet and adequate fluids
11. restriction of visiting to close family

During the rehabilitation phase in hospital, the patient should be encouraged gradually to increase his level of activity daily.

For example:

Up half an hour a.m. and p.m. day 3 post infarction
Up one hour a.m. and p.m. on day 4
Up two hours a.m. and p.m. on day 5
Up as able with rest p.m., walk around bed day 6
Walk to toilet and dayroom day 7

The above is an example of a régime. You could use this, or any with which you are familiar in answer to an examination question.

As the patient becomes more mobile and able to satisfy his own basic needs, the emphasis in care shifts from the physical to the psychological aspect and he and his family will require much support, explanation and counselling in order to come to terms with what has happened. Appropriate health education as identified in the previous section will be necessary and he will require specific information in relation to:

prescribed medication
outpatient attendance
'coronary classes'
his occupation, e.g. a heavy-goods-vehicle driver would lose his special
licence and thus his livelihood

Left ventricular failure

Key facts
1. It is most commonly caused by hypertension or coronary artery disease.

↑ blood pressure → back pressure to left ventricle → hypertrophy of left
ventricle
↓
pulmonary venous congestion ← back pressure to left atrium

2. It may develop gradually or suddenly.
3. Problems patient complains of include dyspnoea, especially orthopnoea and paroxysmal nocturnal dyspnoea; weakness and fatigue.
4. Patient may awaken suddenly with an attack of cardiac asthma:
wheezing; feeling of panic and suffocation; expectorating frothy, sometimes bloodstained, sputum.

Key aspects of nursing management
Initially, priorities of care are directed towards:
1. appropriate position in bed, e.g. sitting up well supported by pillows.
2. positioning bed in easily observable place, preferably in a well-ventilated area near to a window
3. assessment of vital signs, e.g. blood pressure, heart rate, respirations
4. administration of prescribed humidified oxygen, e.g. 40 per cent via
Ventimask
5. administration of prescribed medication: sedatives, e.g. diamorphine,
intravenously to reduce anxiety; diuretics, e.g. frusemide, intravenously
to reduce blood volume/oedema by promoting a diuresis; bronchodilators, e.g. salbutamol via nebulizer, and aminophylline intravenously
6. assistance with chest X-ray and electrocardiogram
7. explanations of treatment and appropriate reassurance to patient and
relatives
8. promote rest and reduce unnecessary exertion, e.g. ensure urinal,
locker, bed table, sputum pot, tissues are within easy reach.
  As condition stabilizes, specific aspects of care include:

1. regular monitoring of vital signs
2. accurate fluid balance record
3. assessment of effect of medication
4. continued explanations and reassurance to patient and relatives
5. continued promotion of rest and sleep with gradual mobilization
6. encouragement or assistance to change position in bed to relieve pressure
7. assistance with hygiene needs as appropriate, e.g. face and hands wash, mouth care.

Congestive cardiac failure

Key facts
1. Failure of the right and left ventricles associated with the retention of fluid in either the lungs or peripheral tissue or both
2. Usually occurs in patients with pulmonary congestion due to left ventricular failure
3. Problems the patient complains of include, dyspnoea; orthopnoea; weight gain (due to fluid retention); generalized oedema; coolness of extremities; anxiety and fear. There may be associated abdominal pain due to 'congestion' of the liver with blood.

Key aspects of nursing management
The care should be directed at the patient's specific problems with an emphasis on reducing the workload on the heart. This includes:
1. appropriate positioning and relief of dyspnoea as for left ventricular failure, *but* if lung disease is present the prescribed oxygen will be of a lower concentration, e.g. 26 per cent.
2. promotion of rest by ensuring that unnecessary physical exertion is avoided, e.g. use of commode; provision of urinal, easy accessibility of bed, locker and possessions; help with washing, hygiene needs, changing of position.
3. relief and prevention of oedema by administration of prescribed medication and monitoring of effects, e.g. digoxin – which slows the heart rate and increases the myocardial contraction. This increases cardiac output; decreases venous pressure and thus promotes diuresis by allowing better perfusion of the kidneys. It is important to observe for side effects due to toxicity and these include cardiac arrhythmias especially bradycardia; anorexia, nausea and vomiting – and frusemide – which produces an effective diuresis by interfering with the reabsorption of sodium in the loop of Henle. It is important to tell the patient about the

rapid action of this drug and to ensure that a urinal or commode is easily available for use. It is also necessary to observe the patient for any evidence of urinary retention, dehydration, hypokalaemia or circulatory collapse as the latter can occur as a result of too rapid a diuresis. Potassium supplements may be prescribed to counteract the hypokalaemia.

The effectiveness of the therapy should be monitored by maintaining an accurate fluid balance chart and daily weighing.

Salt restriction and fluid restriction may also be prescribed by the doctor as may other drugs to help increase cardiac output and promote diuresis and you should ensure that you are aware of the effects of those used commonly in your hospital.

4. Relief of anxiety by adequate explanations of treatment and care as well as allowing time to listen to the patient's fears and worries, and offering reassurance as appropriate. This includes involving the patient's family. Special attention should be paid to the patient at night if he is experiencing paroxysmal nocturnal dyspnoea. Administration of prescribed mild sedatives or analgesia if the patient is experiencing pain will also help to reduce his anxiety.

5. Health education advice should include:

(a) avoiding over-exertion and having a regular daily rest

(b) following an appropriate (not excessive) exercise programme

(c) avoidance of emotional stress

(d) being aware of the actions and side effects of the prescribed medications and appreciating the need to take the drugs as prescribed and to seek help if any side effects occur

(e) complying with dietary instructions, e.g. low sodium, and being aware of which foods to avoid

(f) stopping smoking

(g) avoiding extremes of temperature.

Subacute bacterial endocarditis

Key facts

1. This is infection of the endocardium, often the aortic valve.

2. The commonest infecting organism is *Streptococcus viridans*.

3. Problems the patient complains of include pyrexia (low grade), anorexia, weight loss, increasing tiredness, sweating and vague joint pains.

4. Small emboli can break off from the vegetative growth and pass into the circulation where they characteristically cause small haemorrhages, e.g. under fingernails.

5. Major emboli can become lodged in any organ with serious conse-quences, e.g. in the brain causing a stroke.

Key aspects of nursing management
1. Quiet, well-ventilated position in the ward
2. Psychological support, explanations, reassurance about long period in hospital
3. Light bedcovers and appropriate care relating to pyrexia, e.g. frequent washes, changes of pyjamas, tepid sponging, fanning if necessary
4. Promotion of rest and reduction of unnecessary exertion
5. Prevention of complications associated with bed rest
6. Care of intravenous infusion/cannula and administration of prescribed antibiotics intravenously. This may be for four to six weeks, thus preven-tion of infection and care of the intravenous site are very important, e.g. observation for signs of inflammation; strict adherence to intravenous injection policy
7. Observations for evidence of emboli, haemorrhage or deterioration in condition
8. Education on avoiding infection and the need for antibiotic cover prior to dental extractions or surgery in the future.

Cardiac arrest

As a student you would be expected to be able to identify when cardiac arrest has occurred, describe the action that would be taken to resuscitate the patient and other nursing responsibilities. You would not be expected to be familiar with the details of the medical treatment.

Key facts
Cardiac arrest is indicated by:
1. loss of consciousness
2. no carotid or femoral pulse
3. ceasing of respiration
4. cold, clammy skin
5. dilatation of pupils which occurs in less than one minute
6. grey or cyanosed colour
7. loss of muscle tone.

Key aspects of nursing management
The nursing aim is to restore oxygenated blood and maintain circulation until help arrives.

In answer to a question about the actions you take on discovering a cardiac arrest, the details may be slightly different depending on the hospital policy with which you are familiar, but the sequence of action and responsibilities should be the same.

1. Alert cardiac resuscitation team and note time.
2. Place patient on a firm surface in a supine position with neck extended.
3. Ensure a clear airway.
4. Give a sharp blow to the chest. If this is unsuccessful in restoring cardiac output, commence external cardiac massage and artificial respiration.
5. Ensure cardiac arrest trolley, other appropriate equipment, e.g. suction apparatus, oxygen, are available at the bedside.
6. Screen the bed area and remove locker, chair or other items which may obstruct or impede the actions of the resuscitation team.
7. Assist medical staff with intubation, defibrillation and administration of drugs as requested. Keep an accurate record of the drugs and doses which the doctor gives.

Other specific nursing responsibilities which would continue while the resuscitation was in progress include:

1. ensuring other patients are reassured as necessary and not neglected.
2. informing the next of kin of the patient's condition or ensuring that a nurse takes them to a quiet room and remains with them if they are already on the ward.

If the resuscitation is successful, then ensure that:

1. one nurse is allocated specifically to care for the patient.
2. if requested, arrangements are made to transfer the patient to the coronary care unit.
3. all emergency equipment and drugs are checked and restocked as necessary.
4. the next of kin are able to discuss the events with a senior nurse and that the doctor also explains about the patient's condition to them.

Hypertension

The recording of blood pressure measurements is something that most nurses carry out frequently. It is vital that you understand the importance of doing this and the possible effects of increased blood pressure on an individual. You must also be aware of the advice you can give a patient to help him reduce his blood pressure as well as being able to explain to him about the medication he has been prescribed by the doctor.

Remember that very few patients are admitted to hospital *solely* for treatment of hypertension. The majority are managed without the need for admission by good health education advice and medical treatment.

Key facts

1. *Essential* hypertension is hypertension of which there is no known cause and this affects approximately 90 per cent of all hypertensive patients.
2. Factors thought to be associated with causing hypertension include:
(a) familial tendency
(b) stress, anxiety and other emotional disturbances
(c) obesity
(d) stimulatory drugs including excessive caffeine, nicotine.
3. Hypertension is usually defined as a diastolic pressure persistently greater than 90 mm Hg and a systolic pressure persistently greater than 150 mm Hg. Blood pressure measurements normally vary with regard to:
age
weight
before or after exercise
whether taken during the night or in the daytime
degree of anxiety about procedure.
4. Physiological factors involved in controlling blood pressure include:
(a) higher centres in the brain
(b) sympathetic nervous system
(c) adreno-cortical secretions
(d) renin-angiotensin system
(e) other factors associated with Na^+ and H_2O balance.
5. Drug treatment includes:
(a) diuretics, e.g. spironolactone
(b) β blockers, e.g. propranolol
(c) combined α and β blockers, e.g. labetalol
(d) vasodilators, e.g. hydralazine, methyldopa.

Key aspects of nursing management

1. You should ensure you are familiar with the dosage and effects of above drugs by reference to a suitable text (see p. 152).
2. When recording lying and standing blood pressure always record the in-lying position first. A slight decrease in diastolic and increase in systolic is normal when moving from a lying to standing position.
3. Factors to consider when advising hypertensive patients about controlling their illness include:

(a) regularly taking the medication and being aware of its effects
(b) reducing stress in their lifestyles as far as possible
(c) reducing Na$^+$ intake by avoiding, for example, processed foods, added salt
(d) encouraging regular, but not excessive exercise
(e) reducing weight if obese
(f) possible involvement in relaxation therapy or biofeedback techniques
(g) specific advice relating to identified problems in the particular individual, e.g. support and help to cope with his marital/financial difficulties
(h) health education relating to an identified primary cause, e.g. cardiovascular disease
(i) uncontrolled hypertension can result in:
   (i) cerebrovascular accidents
   (ii) heart failure
   (iii) renal failure.

10.5. Care of patients having surgery

Arterial

It is unlikely that you would be asked to describe nursing care of a patient following major arterial surgery, e.g. repair of a ruptured aortic aneurysm. Key notes relating to care of patients undergoing bypass grafting are included below. You should also be able to discuss the factors associated with peripheral vascular disease (see pp. 156–7) and relate these to the care of a patient requiring an amputation. Care of patients needing amputation is included in this section because many amputations are performed on patients who suffer from problems associated with arterial insufficiency, e.g. intermittent claudication; rest pain; ulceration; cold extremities; local venous collapse; gangrene; absent or weak distal pulses.

Bypass grafts

Key aspects of nursing management
1. *Preoperative*:
(a) Accurate assessment of patient with regard to potential postoperative problems, e.g. due to smoking
(b) Preparation of patient for and assistance with medical investigations, e.g. arteriogram
(c) Routine preoperative preparation (see Chapter 7)
(d) Specific   preparation   related   to   particular   surgical   procedure,

e.g. pubic and full leg shave if prior to femoral-popliteal bypass graft using long saphenous vein

(e) Ensuring surgeon's markings are not removed

(f) Teaching (with physiotherapist) of the exercises necessary postoperatively.

2. *Postoperative*:

(a) Routine postoperative care (Chapter 7)

(b) Specific observations relating to the accurate recording of pulses in the leg and feet (if femoral-popliteal bypass); evidence of 'mottling' or other colour changes and associated temperature changes in the limb

(c) Encouraging patient to carry out exercises which were taught preoperatively to promote circulation

(d) Elevating the legs initially on pillows to reduce oedema

(e) Protecting limb from pressure and promoting easy observation by use of bedcradle

(f) Observing Redivac drains for type, quality of discharge (usually removed after forty-eight hours)

(g) Promoting adequate fluids

(h) Mobilizing in accordance with local surgeon's policy

(i) Health education advice prior to discharge.

Amputation

Key aspects of nursing management

1. *Preoperative*:

(a) Adequate psychological preparation relating to the operation, postoperative care, patient's expectations, fear, anxieties. This should involve all multidisciplinary team members who will be involved in the patient's care

(b) Administration of prescribed medications, e.g. analgesia, antibiotics, and assessment of effect

(c) Teaching patient (with the physiotherapist) about specific exercises to strengthen muscles, lessening the risk of postoperative problems

(d) Ensuring that specific medical tests have been completed and results are available, e.g. haemoglobin, full blood count, grouping and cross-match

(e) Promotion of appropriate diet and adequate fluids

(f) Routine care (see Chapter 7).

2. *Postoperative*:

(a) Immediate and routine care (see Chapter 7)

(b) Care of pain and phantom pains

(c) Observations of vital signs and wound for evidence of haemorrhage

(d) Care of stump, e.g. for an above-knee amputation this would include use of bedcradle, bandaging, sandbags, drawsheet, firm mattress; help with moving; lying prone for half an hour at least twice a day to prevent flexion deformity. Care relating to Redivacs, which are removed after forty-eight hours; sutures removed after ten to fourteen days

(e) Teaching and supervision about exercises, early ambulation, getting up into wheelchair or walking with crutches

(f) Prostheses: fitting; referral to specialist unit

(g) Psychological support relating to altered body image, work, legal worries

(h) Encouraging patient to do things for himself and discuss the amputation

(i) Awareness of patient's need to experience grief reaction (see Chapter 19, p. 294)

(j) Arrangement of appropriate community support (see Chapter 4)

(k) General care relating to problems associated with immobility, potential infection.

N.B. Many patients requiring surgery for peripheral vascular disease are in an older age group and more prone to general complications as a result of their age and general physical condition. You should ensure that you take this into account if your examination answer relates to an elderly person.

Vascular

The points to include in the management of a gravitational ulcer are included in the specimen answer on pp. 18–21, Chapter 1. The sections below only contain points relating to the specific care associated with surgery of varicose veins and haemorrhoids. You would also be expected to know the health education topics which should be included when advising patients who have phlebitis and chronic venous problems of the lower limb, for example,

1. importance of washing feet on a daily basis and ensuring that they are properly dried

2. correct method of cutting toenails – straight across, and after a bath

3. importance of exercise to promote good circulation

4. wearing comfortable shoes

5. avoiding extremes of temperature

6. stopping smoking.

The examiner would also expect you to be able to describe the normal structure of a vein and relate this to the changes associated with varicosities.

Varicose veins

Key facts and associated specific nursing management

1. Varicose veins are abnormally dilated veins.
2. They most commonly occur in lower limbs due to weakness in the walls of the veins.
3. Problems associated with them include aching, tiredness, night cramps, disfigurement. If untreated this can lead to oedema and thus ulceration because of the failure of the calf muscle pump and the resultant venous stasis.
4. Initial advice includes the wearing of elastic stockings, reducing weight if necessary and encouraging exercise. The wearing of constricting clothes, e.g. tight socks, sitting with legs crossed and standing still should be discouraged as these result in increasing the venous pressure and thus the degree of varicosity.
5. If this fails, or is inappropriate, then a sclerotic agent to cause venous fibrosis may be injected.
6. There is no specific nursing preparation prior to ligation and stripping of varicose veins other than that identified in Chapter 7. The nurse must however ensure any marks made by the surgeon on the affected limb are not removed prior to surgery.
7. Postoperatively, specific priorities include observation for signs of haemorrhage, adequate pain relief in the form of analgesia and ensuring a comfortable position. Early ambulation is important and advice as in 4 above should be reiterated. The leg should be kept elevated when sitting. Aseptic wound care should be practised to reduce the risk of infection.

Haemorrhoids

Key facts and associated specific nursing management

1. Haemorrhoids are varicose veins occurring in the submucosa of the anal canal.
2. They can be caused by chronic constipation, pregnancy and inappropriate use of purgatives.
3. Problems associated with them include bleeding on defaecation, itching and pain.
4. Initial advice includes avoidance of straining, promotion of good hygiene, suitable diet to prevent constipation, e.g. including bran.
5. If this fails, they can be treated by injection of a sclerosing agent or haemorrhoidectomy.

6. There is no specific *preoperative* preparation other than that identified in Chapter 7. It is however important that the bowel is empty prior to surgery and that the perineal area is shaved.

7. Specific *postoperative* management includes observation for signs of haemorrhage (remember, this may not be apparent as bleeding via the anus because a pack will be *in situ*), e.g. increasing pulse rate, restlessness and, eventually, falling blood pressure; adequate pain relief especially prior to removal of the pack in a saline bath. Early mobilization should be encouraged and the patient may experience difficulty voiding initially unless allowed to get up. Care to ensure that constipation does not occur is very important and an appropriate diet and a good fluid intake should be encouraged. Use of prescribed laxatives may also assist in prevention of this problem.

8. Dietary and hygiene advice should be given prior to discharge which is normally when there is no evidence of bleeding and the bowels have been opened normally.

10.6. Specimen R.G.N. questions

Q.1. Mr Hughes, aged 82 years, lives alone and is very independent. He is admitted at 03.00 hours, and is very dyspnoeic, cyanosed, cold and clammy. A diagnosis of left ventricular failure is made.

(a) Describe the nursing care and management Mr Hughes will require on his admission and for the rest of the night. 80%

(b) What preparations should be made prior to Mr Hughes's discharge home? 20%

Final R.G.N. paper, English and Welsh National Board, January 1985

Q.2. Mrs Joan Parkes, a 70-year-old widow, is admitted to a medical ward with severe congestive cardiac failure. She is accompanied by her two granddaughters.

Give a detailed account of the nursing measures necessary to alleviate the likely problems which Mrs Parkes may experience. 100%

Final R.G.N. paper, English and Welsh National Board, May 1985

10.7. Sample question and answer

Q. John Murphy, a 43-year-old company executive, is admitted to a medical ward following an attack of angina.

(a) Discuss the information you would need to obtain during the nursing assessment in order to plan his care appropriately.   70%

(b) What advice would you give Mr Murphy to help him to manage his angina when he is discharged?   30%

(a) Your discussion should include:
1. *Information about the pains*
(a) When do the attacks occur?
(b) What are they associated with? – exercise, eating, anxiety?
(c) How long do they last and how frequent are they?
(d) Where is the pain? Does it radiate elsewhere?
(e) What type of pain is it – stabbing, short, continuous, dull?
(f) Details of this particular episode of pain.
2. *Physical assessment*
(a) Recording of blood pressure for evidence of abnormality
(b) Recording of heart rate, rhythm and noting of abnormalities
(c) Any other physical problems e.g. pain related to eating, which may be indicative of an ulcer?
(d) Difficulty with hearing
(e) Problems associated with his bowel movements
(f) Is he overweight?
(g) Is he taking medication? – if so what? When? Has he informed the doctor?
3. *Social psychological assessment*
(a) What is his family/marital status?
(b) Where are his relatives? Is he away from home?
(c) Do they need contacting?
(d) Is he anxious? Why? Does he understand what is wrong and why he is here?
(e) Assess which 'risk factors' are appropriate in his case, e.g. smoking, stress, long working hours, personality type.
   As the answer is a discussion you should indicate how this information can be used in planning his care, e.g. if he suffers from constipation it would be important to ensure that his care plan included dietary advice, encouragement with fluids and administration of prescribed laxatives to avoid him having to 'strain' when defaecating.

Knowledge about the occurrence and type of pain would allow you to help him avoid precipitating factors and to be ready if particular events brought on the pain, e.g. a visit from his family. You would also be better equipped to assess the pain and the effect of medication, e.g. glyceryl trinitrate.

A knowledge of the risk factors allows you to give him appropriate specific counselling and support.

(*b*) Your advice should include:

1. How to deal with an angina attack including details of medications he will have been prescribed and how and when to take them, as well as advice about what to do if they do not work within a short space of time.

2. Preventive measures to avoid an attack, e.g. avoidance of heavy lifting; an appropriate exercise régime; adequate rest periods; stopping smoking; trying to reduce emotionally stressful situations; trying to eat and work regularly and not excessively; avoidance of cold where possible.

10.8. Multiple choice questions

Q.1. Which one of the following is responsible for the pain in angina?
(*a*) *decreased flow of blood through the pulmonary artery*
(*b*) *decreased flow of blood through the myocardium*
(*c*) *increased blood pressure*
(*d*) *arteriosclerosis.*

The pain experienced in angina is due to the lack of oxygen available for use by the myocardial cells; (*b*) is thus the correct answer. It is likely that the patient may suffer from hypertension and have arteriosclerosis but neither of these in themselves is responsible for the pain. Decreased blood-flow through the pulmonary artery is in itself not going to cause pain although it may cause other circulatory and oxygenation problems.

Q.2. Which one of the following mechanisms is most significant in the formation of oedema due to congestive cardiac failure?
(*a*) *high venous pressure*
(*b*) *retention of sodium via the kidney tubule*
(*c*) *decreased blood pressure in the capillaries*
(*d*) *permeability of the capillaries to protein.*

All of the above except (*c*) are associated with the formation of oedema. (*c*) is incorrect because it is an *increase* in blood pressure in the capillaries which is associated with oedema formation. (*b*) is associated with disorders relating to aldosterone production and is not a significant cause of oedema in congestive cardiac failure. Permeability of the capillaries to protein occurs when there is a lack of oxygen in the body and the capillary walls are damaged allowing protein to pass into the tissue spaces. This is associated with congestive cardiac failure but is not the *most* significant mechanism. (*a*) is correct because the major mechanism responsible for oedema in congestive cardiac failure is the high venous pressure and associated stasis.

Q.3. Which one of the following is the antidote for warfarin?
(*a*) *protamine sulphate*
(*b*) *vitamin D*
(*c*) *vitamin K*
(*d*) *propantheline.*

The correct answer is (*c*), as (*a*) is the antidote for heparin; (*b*) is associated with calcium metabolism and (*d*) is an antispasmodic drug.

11. Care of patients with endocrine disorders

11.1. Introduction

This chapter considers the care patients with specific endocrine disorders require. A good knowledge of the physiology of these glands is important in order to understand the problems that the patient may develop and thus be able to plan his care appropriately.

Care of patients with ovarian disorders is discussed in Chapter 15, and related anatomy and physiology can be found in Chapter 9, *Penguin Masterstudies: Biology*.

Key words

An *endocrine* gland is a ductless gland which secretes its products directly into the bloodstream. The chemical substances secreted in this way are called *hormones*.

11.2. The pituitary gland

This is the major endocrine gland in the body.
It consists of an anterior lobe, the *adenohypophysis*, a posterior lobe, the *neurohypophysis* and a small intermediate lobe. It is attached to the *hypothalamus*. The posterior lobe has neural connections with the hypothalamus while the anterior lobe has vascular connections.

The *neurohypophysis* secretes two important hormones:
1. Vasopressin (antidiuretic hormone) which stimulates the reabsorption

of water from the fluid in the collecting ducts of the nephrons in the kidney by increasing permeability of the cells to water and

2. oxytocin which acts on the smooth muscle cells that line the ducts of the breasts causing them to contract and milk to be ejected at the nipple of a lactating female.

The *adenohypophysis* secretes six major hormones:

1. adrenocorticotrophic hormone (adrenocorticotrophin, A.C.T.H.) which stimulates the adrenal cortex to produce cortisol;

2. thyroid-stimulating hormone (thyrotrophin, T.S.H.) which stimulates the thyroid gland to produce T_3 (triiodithyronine) and T_4 (thyroxine);

3. growth hormone (somatotrophin, H.G.H.) which promotes growth in bone, cartilage and soft tissues;

4. prolactin (luteotrophic hormone L.T.H.) which is involved in the initiation and maintenance of lactation;

5. follicle-stimulating hormone (F.S.H.) which stimulates spermatogenesis in men and development of the ovarian follicle in women with associated oestrogen production increase;

6. luteinizing hormone (L.H.) which stimulates the interstitial cells in the testes to produce testosterone and in the female causes the corpus luteum to develop and secrete progesterone.

The production of each of the anterior pituitary hormones is controlled by specific hormones released from the hypothalamus and carried via the portal hypophyseal vessels to the adenohypophysis. See diagram opposite.

11.3. Disorders of the thyroid gland

Key facts

This gland secretes thyroxine (T_4), triiodothyronine (T_3), thyrocalcitonin; 90 per cent of the secretion is T_4.

2. Iodine is necessary for the formation of both T_3 and T_4.

3. T_3 and T_4 are both involved in stimulating the tissue metabolism.

4. Thyrocalcitonin is one of the factors involved in lowering blood calcium levels.

Thyrotoxicosis (*hyperthyroidism*)

This is caused by the overactivity of the thyroid gland as a result of changes in the thyroid tissue, or an increase in T.S.H. secretion from the anterior lobe of the pituitary.

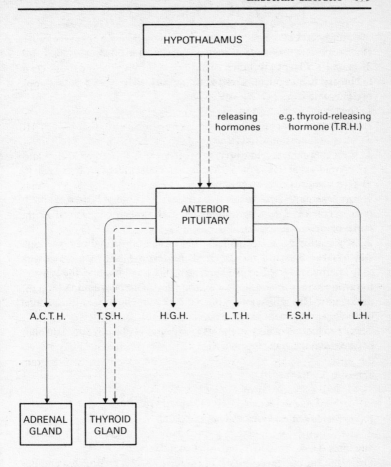

This causes a number of problems for the patient as a result of an increase in the basal metabolic rate.

1. Increased heart rate → palpitations and/or atrial fibrillation
2. Increased heat production → decreased tolerance to heat; increased perspiration
3. Flushed complexion with warm, moist skin
4. Irritability
5. Emotional hyperexcitability
6. Increased appetite associated with weight loss
7. Fine tremor of the hands
8. Changes in bowel habit

9. Amenorrhoea

10. Exophthalmus (protrusion of the eyeballs) is often associated with increased T.S.H. production.

Nursing management is related to the particular problems the patient presents with but would always include:

1. Rest
2. Quiet environment
3. Adequate nutrition and fluids
4. Reducing anxiety and worry.

Three forms of treatment are available for controlling the hyperactivity and thereby providing symptomatic relief.

1. *Drug therapy.* Carbimazole is the drug most commonly used – initially in large doses and then in doses related to the levels of T_3, T_4 and T.S.H. in the blood.

2. *Radioactive iodine.* The patient drinks a solution of radioactive iodine which is then absorbed into the gland and destroys the hyperactive tissue.

It is primarily used in the treatment of carcinoma and the signs of hyperthyroidism should start to reduce after about one month.

3. *Surgery.* This is indicated if the patient cannot be treated by the other methods, or treatment has not succeeded, or malignancy is suspected.

The procedure is usually a subtotal thyroidectomy whereby approximately five-sixths of the gland is removed.

Specific preoperative care

1. Medical drug treatment:
(a) carbimazole to reduce effects of hyperthyroidism;
(b) iodine to reduce vascularity of the gland.

2. Good nutritional intake, e.g. increased carbohydrates, protein and vitamins. Avoid tea, coffee and other stimulants.

3. Ensure the patient is nursed in as quiet an area as possible and has adequate rest.

4. Explain treatment and investigations: C.X.R. (chest X-ray); E.C.G. (electrocardiograph); blood tests; and discuss planned postoperative care.

5. Reduce anxiety/hyperactivity by talking to the patient and trying to help the patient relax.

All normal preoperative preparation would be carried out (see Chapter 7) prior to surgery.

Specific postoperative care

It is vitally important to be aware of the potential complications of this operation and include them in your care. For example,

1. Risk of *obstruction to airway* due to oedema of the glottis or haematoma formation causing pressure on the trachea.

Action: Nurse in semi-prone position until conscious; when conscious nurse in semi-Fowlers position with head well supported with pillows; record respiratory rate half-hourly and observe for any signs of difficulty in breathing, or evidence of cyanosis.

2. Risk of *haemorrhage* following surgery.

Action: Observe wound dressing and also the sides and back of the neck for signs of bleeding. Observe the amount of drainage in the wound Redivac bottle. Record pulse and blood pressure half-hourly. Ask patient to tell you if he experiences any feeling of pressure at the incision site.

If haemorrhage does occur causing obstruction, remove the clips, position the patient on his side and obtain medical assistance.

3. Risk of *tetany* (decrease in blood calcium levels) which occurs if the parathyroid glands were damaged.

Action: Observe for spasms in the hands and feet (carpopedal spasm). Observe for general muscular twitching. Report either to medical staff so that calcium can be prescribed for the patient.

4. Risk of *damage to the recurrent laryngeal nerve* which may lead to respiratory problems or result in the patient having voice changes.

Action: Ensure the patient does not talk too much in the immediate postoperative period. Note any changes in the patient's voice. (N.B. Some hoarseness may occur and this will normally resolve itself within a few days.)

5. *Thyroid crisis*. This is when a sudden increase of thyroxine secreted into the bloodstream occurs.

Action: Monitor temperature regularly for signs of sudden pyrexia. Observe patient for other signs of an increase in metabolic rate, e.g. sweating, tachycardia.

Other points to include are:

1. Difficulty in swallowing – give liquid or semi-solid food
2. Sore throat – encourage fluids and give lozenges/ice cubes to suck
3. Help with movement in bed especially if I.V.I. is *in situ*
4. Regular analgesia – intramuscularly initially
5. Up out of bed on first day postoperatively
6. Drains removed after forty-eight hours
7. Clips removed three to four days postoperatively
8. Discharged home fifth day postoperatively.

Hypothyroidism

When this is present at birth it leads to *cretinism*. When the deficiency occurs in later life it is called *myxoedema*. The problems the patient complains of initially include:
1. Tiredness and lethargy
2. Hair loss, brittle nails and dry skin
3. Menstrual disturbances and loss of libido
4. Constipation.

If the problem is not recognized then the basal metabolic rate slows down further causing

decreased temperature

decreased heat rate

increased weight.

The patient's skin becomes thickened and the face mask-like in appearance. Speech becomes slow as do other cerebral processes.

The treatment is to replace the thyroxine with oral tablets. In adults, this is curative. In children, growth will already have been permanently damaged unless diagnosis was made at birth.

When planning care for these patients their major problem will be lethargy and therefore their inability to care for themselves adequately in relation to the problems identified.

As they will not metabolize drugs quickly, great care should be used if sedative drugs (e.g. night sedation) are given to them.

During the winter elderly patients can develop a myxoedema coma with convulsions and decreased blood pressure, temperature and heart rate. In this event the nursing management will be initially directed towards care of an unconscious patient (see section 8.5, p. 121, for details).

11.4.   Disorders of the parathyroid glands

Key facts

1. There are four glands embedded in the thyroid gland.
2. They produce parathyroid hormone (P.T.H.).
3. P.T.H. is a major factor in the maintenance of plasma calcium levels.
4. It acts on the kidney, bone and gastrointestinal tract to enable an increase in calcium retention by the body to occur.

Hypoparathyroidism

This occurs if too much tissue is removed surgically, or atrophy has occurred to the gland.

It causes a decrease in calcium levels and an increase in phosphorus levels in the blood; and it causes *tetany*.

The patient is likely to complain of:
1. carpopedal spasm
2. numbness, tingling cramps
3. general muscular twitching.

If this is not treated the following may then develop:
1. bronchospasm
2. dysphagia
3. cardiac and cerebral problems.

The condition is treated initially by giving intravenous calcium gluconate.

Nursing management
This should include:
1. providing a quiet environment for the patient, e.g. a side room because of his increased neuromuscular activity.
2. advice about diet – low phosphorus; high calcium; vitamin D supplements. Milk should be restricted as it contains high phosphorus as well as high calcium.

Hyperparathyroidism

This is caused by overactivity of the gland resulting in the following problems for the patient:
1. fatigue and muscular weakness
2. constipation
3. nausea and vomiting
4. cardiac arrhythmias (with high calcium concentration)
5. renal calculi formation.

The treatment is to remove the abnormal parathyroid tissue.

Preoperative care
This should include:
1. increased fluids (2 to 3 litres per day) to decrease formation of renal stones
2. increased fruit in diet

3. decreased milk in diet
4. encouraging patient to be active as much as possible.

Postoperative care
As for thyroidectomy.

11.5. Disorders of the adrenal glands

Key facts

1. There are two distinct parts of each gland.
2. The inner area is called the *medulla*.
3. The outer area is called the *cortex*.
4. Each part produces different endocrine secretions.

The *medulla* produces the catecholamines: adrenaline and noradrenaline. These hormones are active in stressful situations, e.g. anger, fear, ↓ blood sugar, ↓ blood pressure, ↓ cerebral oxygenation. The effect they produce is a sympathetic nervous system effect. For example:

1. dilatation of pupils
2. dilatation of coronary arteries and bronchioles
3. constriction of peripheral blood vessels
4. mobilization of glycogen for conversion to glucose
5. ↑ basal metabolic rate.

The *cortex* produces

1. glucocorticoids
2. mineralocorticoids
3. sex hormones.

1. The main glucocorticoid is cortisol (hydrocortisone). Its production is stimulated by the release of adrenocorticotrophic hormone (A.C.T.H.) from the anterior lobe of the pituitary.

It is involved in regulating the metabolism of fats, carbohydrates and proteins in such a way that it causes a rise in blood glucose levels. It also has anti-inflammatory and anti-allergic effects.

2. The main mineralocorticoid is aldosterone and its primary function is in maintaining the sodium chloride balance in the body. It does this by ↑ sodium absorption in the renal tubules.

3. The effect of sex hormone secretion in normal circumstances compared with the effect of the hormones produced by the gonads is of little significance.

Diseases related to the adrenal glands

Addison's Disease

In this case there is underactivity of the gland.

The problems caused to the patient may include:

1. ↓ blood sugar leading to weakness and lethargy
2. ↓ blood sodium levels leading to ↓ blood volume and water loss
3. nausea and vomiting.

The treatment is to give hydrocortisone for its glucocorticoid effect and fludrocortisone for its mineralocorticoid effect.

An Addisonian crisis is an emergency as the patient will be shocked, i.e. ↓ blood pressure: ↑ pulse: ↑ respiration, fever (if precipitated by infection). Initial treatment is directed towards restoring blood circulation, fluid and electrolyte balance, and treating the precipitating cause.

Nursing management

Education of the patient about his drug therapy is an important aspect. He should be informed as to:

1. what the side effects are
2. what to do in stressful situations
3. what to do if he has an infection
4. the importance of taking the medication as prescribed.

(N.B. The side effects of steroids will cause the patient the same problems as overactivity of the gland.)

Cushing's Syndrome

This is due to overactivity of the adrenal gland. The patient may complain of some or all of the following:

moon face – fat and rounded

thin arms and legs – muscle wasting and weakness

large obese abdomen

tendency to bruise and purple striae on the skin

increased body and facial hair

irregular menstruation and loss of libido

generalized weakness and lethargy

mood changes

some development of masculine features in women, e.g. deep voice.

Medical treatment is to give metyrapone which reduces cortisol synthesis and dexamethasone as replacement therapy.

Important nursing measures include *diet* – high protein, low sodium, low carbohydrate; and *psychological support* about physical appearance, mood changes, depression, 'sexual change'.

If the illness is due to actual adrenal disease as opposed to the effects of steroid therapy, the surgical treatment possible is adrenalectomy.

Specific preoperative care
1. Increased protein diet
2. Drug therapy: metyrapone and dexamethasone

(N.B. Patients with high cortisol levels have a tendency to bleed. Thus, it is very important this is reduced prior to surgery and reduction may take several weeks of drug treatment.)

Specific postoperative care
1. Initially nurse semi-prone until conscious and then with only one pillow.
2. Half-hourly blood pressure and pulse recordings as sudden hypotension may occur.
3. Administer intravenous hydrocortisone initially
4. Give potassium supplements.
5. Oral cortisone and fludrocortisone can be given after a few days.
6. When patient is lying flat ensure two-hourly change of position.
7. Encourage leg exercises and deep breathing.
8. By day 3 postoperatively, if blood pressure is stable start gradually to sit patient up, at first in bed and then in a chair.
9. Monitor blood pressure four-hourly for postural hypotension.

(N.B. Normal postoperative surgical care is required: care of nasogastric tube, intravenous infusion, wound drains.)

Prior to discharge
1. Educate patient and family about taking medication regularly and consistently.
2. Give patient steroid treatment card and ask him to carry it at all times.
3. Suggest patient obtains a Medic Alert bracelet.
4. Advise patient to avoid extreme fatigue, excitement or change in temperature.
5. Tell patient to contact general practitioner if he feels weak, nauseous, vomits or has a rise in temperature.
6. Explain that it takes some months to recover fully and if he has a bilateral adrenalectomy he will *always* require steroid therapy.

Investigations carried out on patients with adrenal disease include: blood tests for cortisol; A.C.T.H. levels; twenty-four-hour urine collection for 17-hydroxycorticosteroids.

11.6. The pancreas and diabetes mellitus

The pancreas

The pancreas has both *exocrine* and *endocrine* functions. Most of the gland is involved in the exocrine secretion of pancreatic juice.

The endocrine function is the production of two hormones involved in blood glucose maintenance. These hormones are produced from groups of cells known as the *islets of Langerhans*.

There are two types of cell:
1. α produce *glucagon* which raises the blood glucose level
2. β produce *insulin* which lowers the blood glucose level.

Insulin is the only hormone to lower blood glucose levels directly whereas many hormones can act to raise it.

Diabetes mellitus

This disorder is the result of a failure of the β cells to produce significant quantities of insulin.

The main effect of insulin is that it increases the ability of glucose to enter the cells, especially muscle and adipose tissue, and overall it promotes the storage of fats, carbohydrates and proteins.

There are two main types of diabetes mellitus.
1. Insulin dependent (I.D.D.M.). This is sometimes referred to as 'juvenile onset', as it is normally diagnosed during childhood. It is characterized by a sudden onset associated with rapid weight loss, polyuria and polydipsia leading to ketoacidosis.
2. Non-insulin dependent (N.I.D.D.M.). This is sometimes referred to as 'maturity onset' as it normally starts after the age of 40 and is gradual or insidious. It is often associated with tiredness, gradual weight loss and possible nocturia. Often the diagnosis is made when the patient presents for treatment of another problem such as cardiac or renal disease, vascular ulcers, pruritis, visual irregularities.

Important factors associated with the development of diabetes include:
Family history
Obesity
Early atherosclerosis
Glucose intolerance relating to drug therapy.

Diet

This is an important factor in the management of these patients and a typical balanced diet should contain approximately 50 per cent carbohydrate, 30 per cent fat, 20 per cent protein. The overall calorie restriction would depend upon the patient's weight age and level of activity but would normally be between 1000 to 2000 calories daily.

The carbohydrates in the intake should contain starch, found, for example, in potatoes, pasta, pulses, while carbohydrates containing sugar, such as sweets, honey, and alcohol, should be avoided.

The fat intake should be of vegetable fat origin where possible.

In many N.I.D.D.M. patients, dietary control to reduce calorie intake and regular exercise to utilize glucose are sufficient to control the disease. If this is unsuccessful then drug therapy is necessary.

Oral hypoglycaemic drugs

There are two types:
1. sulphonylureas
2. biguanides.

(a) Sulphonylureas stimulate the release of insulin from the β cells of the islets of Langerhans, e.g. tolbutamide; chlorpropamide; glibenclamide.
(b) Biguanides reduce the absorption of carbohydrate from the gut and enhance glucose uptake by muscle cells, e.g. metformin.

Both groups can only work if some insulin is present. The sulphonyl-ureas have very few side effects while biguanides can cause gastrointestinal problems.

Insulin

All insulin is now standardized in solution of 100 units per ml.

For fast action either soluble or Actrapid insulin is used. For longer action, insulin (*lente*) in combination with zinc is used as this increases the duration of action.

Most diabetics can be controlled by daily injections of a *lente* prep-aration or by injections of soluble insulin prior to meals. The sites for injection should be varied to avoid hypertrophy of the fatty tissue and localized tenderness. Injections are normally given intradermally at right angles to the skin.

Complications of the disease

1. *Hypoglycaemia* (blood glucose level less than 2 mmol L^{-1}). Associated with rapid onset.
Signs:
sweating
tachycardia
tremor

confusion
slurred speech
drowsiness leading to coma.
causes:
too much exercise
too much insulin
insulin not followed by a meal
unstable diabetes due to a secondary cause, e.g. infection following surgery.
Action:
Give oral glucose. If unable to, give intravenous glucose (10 mls 20 per
cent dextrose) or 1 mg glucagon subcutaneously or intramuscularly.
2. *Hyperglycaemia*. Associated with slow onset.
Signs:
polydipsia and polyuria leading to dehydration
vomiting and lethargy
oliguria
Kussmaul respirations (deep and sighing)
drowsiness → coma
Causes:
omission of insulin
resistance to insulin
infection
stress
undiagnosed diabetes.
Action:
Prompt medical treatment is necessary to prevent the patient becoming
comatose. This will include prescribing intravenous insulin; intravenous
potassium chloride, sodium bicarbonate and other electrolytes as appropriate; intravenous fluid replacement 4 to 6 litres in twenty-four hours.
Nursing management:
This should include:
(a) frequent recording of pulse, respirations and blood pressure
(b) regular monitoring of temperature for pyrexia
(c) hourly measurements of urine and testing for glucose and ketones
(d) maintenance of intravenous fluids as prescribed
(e) maintenance of insulin infusion pump as prescribed in relation to
blood glucose levels
(f) recording of central venous pressure.
   Management of the patient also includes treating any precipitating
illness or infection, and unconsciousness if present.

Patient education

This is an important part of nursing management and is often included in questions relating to diabetes.

When explaining diabetes to a newly diagnosed patient the following should be taken into account:

age of the patient

family situation

importance of a clear, simple explanation

not using hospital jargon

providing leaflets/books

encouraging questions

repeating information at a later date.

Subjects which must be included when preparing a patient for return home are:

1. Understanding of hypoglycaemia and how to avoid it

2. Understanding of hyperglycaemia and the importance of consulting a doctor if an infection develops

3. The ability to test urine accurately or to make accurate blood glucose estimations

4. The ability to store correctly and calculate dosage of insulin

5. The ability to give injections correctly and to understand the importance of rotating the sites

6. Understanding of dietary régime and its relation to exercise and insulin requirements

7. Where to gain further advice from, e.g. the British Diabetic Association.

11.7. Specimen R.G.N. question

Q. Miss Carol Rush, a 31-year-old beautician, is admitted to hospital following medical treatment for thyrotoxicosis. She is to undergo partial thyroidectomy.

(a) Identify the specific physical preoperative preparation Miss Rush will require prior to and following her admission, explaining why this is important.

60%

(b) Discuss how Miss Rush's anxiety may be minimized before and after surgery.

40%

R.G.N. paper, English and Welsh National Board, July 1984

11.8. Sample question and answer

Q. Peter Collins, aged 19 years, is admitted to a medical ward in a drowsy state due to ketoacidosis. He was only diagnosed as suffering from diabetes mellitus six weeks ago and is a student at college.

(a) Discuss the possible reasons which may have precipitated this episode of ketoacidosis.   30%

(b) Outline a plan of care for the first six hours in hospital.   70%

(*a*) The discussion must include the following:

1. Infection: has Peter a respiratory or urinary tract infection, or any other source of infection, as this would increase the body's demands for insulin?

2. Exercise: has Peter changed his rest/exercise pattern since going to college so that he now requires more insulin?

3. Diet: is he eating regular meals and having a well-balanced diet? Does he understand the importance of this? Has he been drinking alcohol?

4. Insulin: does he fully understand how to draw up the correct amount of insulin in the syringe and is he administering it properly?

5. Stress: is he under specific stress in relation to college or social/home situation?

(*b*) This is best answered by identifying the problems Peter has or may have in the first six hours and planning care in relation to them.

Actual problems	Nursing action
Dehydration	1. Record hourly urine output. 2. Record fluid intake. 3. Care of intravenous infusion. 4. Monitor central venous pressure if manometer *in situ.* 5. Record blood pressure.
Drowsiness	1. Observe conscious level for signs of change/deterioration. 2. Regulate insulin infusion as prescribed. 3. Test urine for glucose and ketones. 4. Test blood for glucose. 5. Give intravenous fluids and electrolytes as prescribed in relation to blood results. 6. Observe and record respiratory rate.

Potential problems	Nursing action
Obstruction of airway	1. Nurse semi-prone while drowsy.
	2. Ensure suction equipment available near bed in case of need.
	3. Observe and record respiratory rate.
Cardiac arrhythmias	1. Observe cardiac monitor for arrhythmias.
	2. Record heart rate.
	3. Assist with electrocardiogram.
	4. Give intravenous potassium as prescribed.

The answer should concentrate on the above in relation to the first six hours. However, it would also be relevant to include more briefly other aspects of care relating to dry mouth due to dehydration; potential pyrexia due to infection; nausea and/or vomiting.

11.9. Multiple choice questions

Q.1. Which one of the following may a patient with thyrotoxicosis be most likely to suffer from?
(a) *anorexia, dyspnoea and drowsiness*
(b) *tachycardia, loss of weight and anorexia*
(c) *drowsiness, large appetite and weight gain*
(d) *large appetite, loss of weight and tachycardia.*

The correct answer is (d) as all the symptoms are associated with an increased metabolic rate. The patient will have a good appetite but will still lose weight because of increased demands for energy by the body. Drowsiness and weight gain are associated with hypothyroidism and thus (a) and (c) can be eliminated.

Anorexia is not associated with thyrotoxicosis thus (b) can also be eliminated. Dyspnoea is also not normally associated with thyrotoxicosis unless it is secondary to cardiac failure due to increased heart rate.

Q.2. Which one of the following signs will be most prevalent in the event of a thyroid crisis following a partial thyroidectomy?
(a) *twitching of muscles*
(b) *sudden temperature elevation*
(c) *sudden extreme drowsiness*
(d) *falling blood pressure and rising pulse rate.*

The correct answer is (*b*) as a thyroid crisis is associated with a sudden increase in thyroxine secretion into the blood system following surgery thus causing an increase in metabolic rate.

(*a*) is due to tetany associated with parathyroid gland damage.

(*c*) is likely to be due to a neurological problem rather than an increase in thyroxine.

(*d*) is associated with postoperative haemorrhage.

Q.3. Which one of the following is Cushing's Syndrome characterized by:
(*a*) *decreased glucocorticoid secretion*
(*b*) *hypotension*
(*c*) *thick skin*
(*d*) *slow wound healing.*

The correct answer is (*d*) because the increased steroid production interferes with the normal wound-healing process by reducing the normal inflammatory response.

(*a*) is incorrect because an increase in glucocorticoid secretion would be expected due to overactivity of the gland.

(*b*) is incorrect because any change in blood pressure would be an increase due to increased sodium retention.

(*c*) is unrelated to adrenal hormone secretion, although an increase in adipose tissue would occur especially in the abdominal region.

Q.4. Which of the following is the most important observation that should be made on a patient in the immediate postoperative period following an adrenalectomy?
(*a*) *wound site*
(*b*) *urinary output*
(*c*) *blood pressure*
(*d*) *pulse rate.*

The correct answer is (*c*) because there is a risk of a sudden hypotensive episode.

(*a*), (*b*) and (*d*) are also important as with any postoperative care régime but (*c*) is especially important following this operation.

Q.5. Which one of the following represents the most appropriate sequence in the treatment of a diabetic ketoacidotic coma?
(*a*) *intravenous fluids, test urine, glucagon, check blood glucose*
(*b*) *soluble insulin, check blood sugar, test urine, intravenous fluids*

(*c*) *check blood glucose, intravenous fluids, soluble insulin, give potassium supplement*

(*d*) *soluble insulin, intravenous fluids, check blood glucose, test urine.*

The correct answer is (*d*) because as you already know the patient is in a diabetic coma, measuring the blood glucose level is not vital as it will be very high. Thus, giving soluble insulin and fluids is vital followed by regular monitoring of blood glucose and urine ketone levels.

(*a*) is incorrect because glucagon would worsen the situation.

(*b*) and (*c*) are incorrect because the sequence of events does not correspond to the best way of treating this emergency.

12. Care of patients with problems relating to the gastrointestinal tract and other abdominal organs

12.1. Introduction 12.2. Key points relating to anatomy and physiology 12.3. Diet and nutrition 12.4. Principles of abdominal surgical care 12.5. Care of stomas 12.6. Specific care relating to gastrointestinal tract disorders 12.7. Specific care relating to disorders of other organs: the liver; the gall bladder 12.8. Specimen R.G.N. questions 12.9. Sample question and answer

12.1. Introduction

Many of the topics covered in this chapter are those which you should expect to be asked about in an examination as they relate to specific care of patients in areas that all student nurses have gained some experience in. More specialized and less common subjects with which all students would not be familiar are not included in the chapter.

As in other chapters a sound basic knowledge of anatomy and physiology is important in order to understand the reasons why patients experience specific problems and why particular nursing action is taken. You are strongly advised to learn about the appropriate areas identified in 12.2.

The principles relating to abdominal surgical nursing care are identified and those should be applied to the individual patient or situation that you are asked about in an examination question in conjunction with appropriate specific care.

It is important to remember that the changing emphasis in the syllabus indicates that you will be expected to be up to date with current research relating to some of the topics covered, e.g. pain relief. You should have read basic appropriate research such as J. C. Hayward, 'Information as a prescription against pain', Royal College of Nursing, 1975, as well as current papers and relate these to your care.

In the intermediate (interim) examination the longer question may well be related to a topic such as pain or dietary advice and care and you need to read around these subjects to an appropriate depth.

You may also be asked about terminal illness and the nursing care in relation to an abdominal problem, e.g. advanced abdominal carcinoma or liver failure. You should refer to Chapter 9 for the general principles of care but remember to relate the problems and nursing actions to the specific abdominal cause.

Finally, remember that you have cared for many patients following abdominal surgery and with abdominal problems. Try to relate your clinical experience to the question as in this way you are more likely to remember the specific aspects of care that are so important to the patient.

12.2. Key points relating to anatomy and physiology

The gastrointestinal tract

You should ensure that you are familiar with:
1. the functions of the digestive system – ingestion, digestion, absorption, elimination
2. the names and positions of the various parts as well as the associated organs and their roles
3. the structure of a tooth as well as the functions of the different types of teeth
4. the mechanics of eating, swallowing, peristalsis
5. the structure of the stomach including the tissue layers – peritoneum, muscle, submucous, mucous membrane
6. the functions of the stomach and how the structure is related to these functions
7. the role and functions of the different parts of the intestines and the function of specific structures, e.g. villi.

The above are all included in appropriate textbooks and you should refer to these and your lecture notes for relevant details.

The liver

You must be familiar with its anatomical position and general functions, e.g.
1. its role in relation to blood formation – storage of vitamin B_{12}, blood destruction – breakdown of red blood cells into amino acids, iron and bilirubin;

Red blood cell destruction

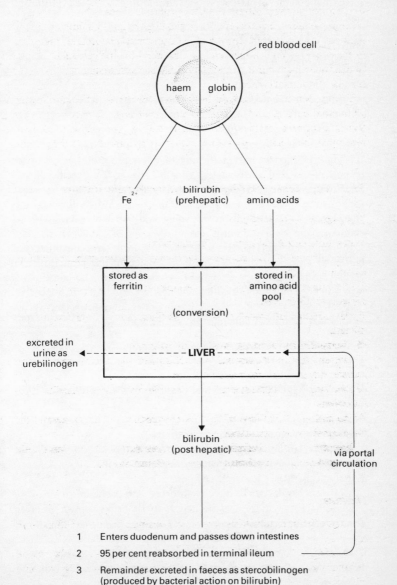

1 Enters duodenum and passes down intestines

2 95 per cent reabsorbed in terminal ileum

3 Remainder excreted in faeces as stercobilinogen
   (produced by bacterial action on bilirubin)

2. the manufacture of plasma proteins and clotting factors, e.g. prothrombin, fibrinogen;
3. its role in food digestion and metabolism, e.g. storage of glycogen; conversion of ammonia to urea; production of bile salts; storage of fat-soluble vitamins, A and D;
4. its role in detoxification of poisons and drugs.

12.3. Diet and nutrition

It is important for the nurse to be able to give appropriate dietary advice to patients as well as to understand the reasons for specific dietary measures being taken in response to specific illnesses. It is also necessary for you to be able to promote good nutrition and healthy eating habits to all age groups – this includes advice you would give to parents and young children in the paediatric wards about prevention of dental caries.

It is thus important for you to be aware of the general constituents of particular types of food, how these are related to our normal dietary needs, and how an excess or inability to absorb particular constituents results in poor nutritional health and illness.

A balanced diet should contain carbohydrates, fats and proteins as well as sufficient supplies of mineral salts, vitamins and water.

Key facts relating to digestion

Digestion is a complex process and you should know the principal points.

Carbohydrates
There are three basic types of carbohydrates:
1. monosaccharides, e.g. glucose, fructose, galactose
2. disaccharides, e.g. sucrose, lactose, maltose
3. polysaccharides, e.g. starch, cellulose.

Monosaccharides can be directly absorbed into the bloodstream.

Disaccharides require enzyme action to be broken down prior to absorption. For example,

$$sucrose \xrightarrow{sucrase} glucose + fructose$$

$$lactose \xrightarrow{lactase} glucose + galactose$$

$$\text{maltose} \xrightarrow{\text{maltase}} \text{glucose}$$

Starch also requires enzyme action. For example,

$$\text{starch} \xrightarrow{\text{amylase}} \text{maltose} \xrightarrow{\text{maltase}} \text{glucose}.$$

Cellulose cannot be absorbed as there is no enzyme present in the digestive system to break it down. It thus contributes bulk to the intestinal contents and promotes peristalsis.

After absorption galactose and fructose are converted to glucose and stored as glycogen or fat.

Fats

Most fat is ingested in the form of triglyceride and is acted upon by pancreatic lipase prior to emulsification by the bile salts:

$$\text{triglyceride} \xrightarrow{\text{lipase}} \underbrace{\text{2-monoglyceride} + \text{free fatty acids}}$$
$$\text{micelles} \xleftarrow{\text{emulsified by bile salts}}$$

Micelles are colloid-sized particles, made up of monoglycerides, free fatty acids and bile salts, and readily able to be absorbed via the microvilli.

Fat-soluble vitamins – A, D, E, K – are incorporated into these micelles to facilitate absorption.

Saturated fatty acids are normally of animal origin.

Unsaturated fatty acids are normally of vegetable origin.

The essential fatty acids which the body must absorb as it is unable to synthesize them are linoleic, linolenic and arachidonic.

Protein

There are approximately twenty different amino acids found in body proteins.

There are eight essential amino acids which must be ingested as they are not synthesized in sufficient quantities in the body.

Protein is necessary for growth and repair of tissues as well as a source of energy.

The breakdown of proteins to amino acids during digestion can be summarized as follows:

in the stomach: protein $\xrightarrow{\text{pepsin}}$ long chain peptides

in the pancreatic juice: $\xrightarrow{\text{trypsin}}$ short chain peptides

in mucosal cells: $\xrightarrow{\text{erepsin}}$ amino acids.

All animal protein contains all essential amino acids.
Most meals contain all the amino acids.

Vitamins

Vitamin A
There are two types: carotene and retinol. Carotene is found in carrots, green vegetables. Retinol is found in fish-liver oil. Both are in butter and cream.

It is necessary to the growth and repair of body tissues especially teeth (enamel) and epithelium and for regeneration of visual purple.

Deficiency results in night blindness, dry skin and eyes, and degeneration in tooth enamel.

Vitamin B complex
This covers many essential vitamins and most are actively involved in providing energy for the body by acting as precursors in the chemical metabolism of carbohydrates, fats and proteins. Most can be found in brewer's yeast, wholegrain cereals or liver and many are produced by intestinal bacteria.

Below are some of the more important individual actions but you should refer to your textbook for further details.
1. B_2 (riboflavin) is important for healthy nails, skin and hair and deficiency can cause mouth ulceration.
2. B_6 (pyridoxine) is necessary for the proper absorption of vitamin B_{12}.
3. B_{12} is necessary for the maturation of erythrocytes (see Chapter 16) and deficiency results in pernicious anaemia.
4. Choline is associated with utilization of fats and cholesterol and deficiency is thought to be associated with increased fatty deposits in the arteries.
5. Folic acid is important in nucleic acid synthesis, cell division and foetal growth.

Vitamin C (Ascorbic acid)
Found in fresh fruit and vegetables.

It has an important role in relation to collagen and facilitates connective tissue formation in scar tissue and aids erythrocyte formation.

It is destroyed by cooking.

Vitamin D
Available naturally from the action of ultraviolet sunlight on the skin or from fish-liver oil as vitamin D_3.

It is available synthetically as vitamin D_2 (calciferol).

It is involved in Ca^{2+} and PO_4^{3-} metabolism.

It is necessary for calcification of bones and teeth in children and a deficit in children results in rickets.

Vitamin K
There are three types: K_1 and K_2 are manufactured in the gastrointestinal tract by bacteria flora; K_3 is synthetic.

Main sources are intestinal flora and green vegetables.

It is essential for formation of prothrombin.

There are other vitamins which are included in the diet but the above are the main ones. You should ensure that you are able to give examples of the types of food which contain appropriate vitamins and be able to explain the need for them.

It may be helpful for you to obtain the information booklets which your hospital dietitian produces for patients as these will indicate to you the foods which are high in mineral salts as well as the relative amounts of carbohydrates, fats and proteins. For example, processed food has a high salt (Na^+) content; fresh fruit juices have a high potassium (K^+) content; milk has a high Calcium (Ca^{2+}) content.

It is important for you to know this in order to give the correct advice to patients who have dietary restrictions or who require general health education advice about their diet.

12.4. Principles of abdominal surgical care

The general principles relating to admission, assessment and pre- and postoperative care as identified in Chapter 7 apply equally to care of patients having abdominal surgery. However, certain key points should always be remembered when planning care for these patients.

Skin preparation
1. Has appropriate skin preparation taken place?
2. Does the area shaved relate correctly to the site of the operation?
3. Has a pre-operation bath been taken?
4. Has any specific skin preparation been used?
5. Should the above be omitted because of the patient's acute pain or cardiovascular status being poor?
6. If the answer to 5 is yes, have the theatre nurses and surgeon been informed?
7. Would the patient have been taken directly to theatre from the accident and emergency department anyway?

Specific preoperative care
1. Does a nasogastric tube need to be passed? Why?
2. Should an intravenous infusion be set up? Why?
3. Have specific tests/investigations been carried out?
4. Has appropriate psychological support been given, if possible, prior to stoma formation, radical abdominal surgery?
5. Is the patient aware of which 'drips and drains' he will have postoperatively?
6. If it is planned that he is to go to the intensive care unit, has this been discussed with him and his family?

'Drips and drains'
1. What intravenous support will he require following the operation, e.g. peripheral line, central line, intravenous cannula for administration of antibiotics?
2. Is it necessary to measure central venous pressure? How frequently?
3. Is the intravenous transfusion for maintenance of hydration, administration of drugs, or to allow a blood transfusion to be given?
4. What drains are there? Are they appropriate to the surgery performed? For example, a Yeates (corrugated drain) would be used for drainage of the secretions from the abdominal cavity and is inserted via a 'stab' wound; a T tube would be used to drain secretions from the common bile duct; A Redivac would be used to drain secretions from the operative area and is usually inserted via the wound incision.
5. How long are the drains left in for?
6. How do you remove them? For example, for corrugated drains, by shortening first.
7. What specific care/observations do the drains require?

Eating and drinking
1. Has the patient had major or minor surgery?
2. Has the bowel been resected, operated on, bruised?
3. Are bowel sounds present?
4. Always commence oral intake with sips of water → more water → tea and then food.
5. Never give fluids/food to patients with *no* bowel sounds.
6. Is there a nasogastric tube *in situ*? Why?
7. Is it being aspirated? How often? What type of drainage? How much? Is it also on continuous drainage?
8. Patients who have had minor abdominal procedures or surgery not involving the bowel should be able to drink within a few hours once they have recovered from the effect of the anaesthetic.
9. Patients who have had major surgery should only commence fluids gradually, when bowel sounds are present and according to medical instructions.
10. Appropriate care to relieve nausea and vomiting.

Elimination
1. Is the patient likely to become constipated due, for example, to immobility, poor diet, analgesia?
2. What action can you take if he does? ↑Fluids; ↑mobility; promote good diet; administer prescribed aperients.
3. Are there difficulties passing urine? Why? Does this relate to the operation, the anaesthetic or both?
4. Observe for signs of retention of urine and report to medical staff.
5. Accurately record fluid input and output.

Pain
1. Ensure *regular* intramuscular pain relief as prescribed during the initial postoperative period.
2. *Do not* wait until the patient is in pain before administering analgesia.
3. Take other measures to promote comfort and relieve pain.
4. Give appropriate analgesia, e.g. not two Panadol, following an abdominoperineal resection.
5. Identify other causes of pain, e.g. retention of urine, constipation, and take action to rectify these.

Wounds
1. Do not inspect unnecessarily.
2. Use strict aseptic technique.

3. Re-dress if required.
4. What types of sutures are there?
5. When should they be removed?
6. For what signs of infection do you observe the wound – inflammation, discharge, redness?
7. Take wound swabs as necessary.

It is also important when considering care of patients following abdominal surgery to include early mobilization in your care plan.

You should also relate the position in bed to the surgery performed, e.g. sit patient up following cholecystectomy to facilitate breathing.

12.5. Care of stomas

Stomas can be formed for a variety of reasons involving different sections of bowel. The principles of care both pre- and postoperatively are the same for either an ileostomy or a colostomy.

Preoperative
Physical preparation is aimed at removing waste material from the bowels so that there is less risk of faecal contamination or damage to the anastomosis and the wound site.

In answer to a question you should describe the specific bowel preparation with which you are familiar as it will vary from hospital to hospital.

An example of a régime might be a low-residue diet for two days followed by clear fluids only on the day prior to surgery. At the same time laxatives, e.g. magnesium sulphate, would be administered regularly to promote diarrhoea. Colonic washouts would also be given on the day prior to surgery and the morning of the operating day.

Psychological preparation is aimed at reducing the anxiety associated with the operation and its effects. This should include:
1. explanation of the surgery and 'what the stoma is'. This can be explained by use of diagrams and/or photographs
2. involvement of family if possible in the discussions
3. development of a trusting relationship by creating an appropriate atmosphere for the patient to ask questions and to give him truthful answers which he can understand
4. early involvement of the stoma therapist
5. opportunity to meet another patient with a stoma if he wishes

6. advice about the appliances and methods of preventing odours
7. allow patient to familiarize himself with the appliances by handling them
8. discuss with patient his fears about his change in body image and sexuality, and counsel accordingly
9. explain to patient and family about the support after the operation.

Postoperative

It is important to be aware of the type of effluent produced by the different stomas in order to give appropriate care, e.g. ileostomy → fluid or paste-like faeces; transverse colostomy → semi-fluid to soft faeces; descending and sigmoid colostomy → soft to solid faeces.

Physical care is directed at:
1. ensuring that the correct size of appliance is used; that it is transparent to allow easy observation and that it can be emptied easily.
2. observing the stoma and skin to ensure they are healthy, and reporting signs of excoriation or infection as well as assessing stoma function.
3. carrying out stoma care in a consistent way with the increasing involvement of the patient so that he can learn to carry out his own stoma care
4. administration of irrigation or suppositories as prescribed.

You should be able to describe how stoma care is carried out in your training hospital, and include reference to appropriate aids, e.g. deodorizers, use of Karaya seals or periostomal wafers, corsets, belts, appliance covers.

Psychological care

This is directed at:
1. continuing discussion of the subjects identified in the preoperative care section
2. allowing patient to experience grief reaction associated with alteration to body image and loss
3. providing opportunities for patient to discuss his fears and anxieties
4. regular counselling from stoma therapist or other appropriate counsellor
5. encouraging patient to increase his responsibility for his colostomy
6. supporting him through occasional setbacks and difficulties
7. preparing him for discharge by ensuring he is confident to physically change his appliance; teaching him about his diet, and ways to adjust it to produce regular faecal evacuation; giving him information about where to get his appliances; how to get them; when to attend outpatients'

department; telephone numbers and addresses of appropriate agencies, e.g. the Ileostomy Association; and community nurse support.

The purpose of the above is to allow the patient to accept his stoma and to have sufficient knowledge to enable him to care for it confidently once he has left the hospital.

12.6. Specific care relating to gastrointestinal problems

Many of the points included in Chapter 7 and 12.3., 12.4. and 12.5. apply to topics covered in this section. Thus, only brief key points are included here.

General points which should always be considered when assessing planning care for patients with gastrointestinal problems include:
1. Pain: where? What type? What causes it? What relieves it?
2. Nausea and vomiting: when does it occur? How much? How often? Do they occur separately?
3. Dietary habits: what type of diet is eaten? How consistent is his weight? Are meals eaten regularly?
4. Eating: are there any mechanical difficulties, e.g. pain on swallowing? Does he feel uncomfortable following a meal? Is there flatulence, belching, heartburn, regurgitation?
5. Elimination: is he constipated or does he suffer from diarrhoea? Are his bowels open regularly? How often? Has this changed recently? Does he take laxatives or other medications? Why? Has he passed blood in his stool?

In addition you should be able to describe the role of the nurse in relation to the appropriate investigations of gastrointestinal function, e.g. gastroscopy; colonoscopy; sigmoidoscopy; barium meal, follow through, enema; observation/collection of stool specimens.

Key points to remember in care of patients with nasogastric tubes
1. Prepare equipment – tube, lubricant, water, syringe, tape.
2. Explain procedure to patient.
3. Prepare patient – sitting up, protection, tissues, screening of bed.
4. Insert lubricated tube – if the patient is allowed to swallow small sips of water this will often help.
5. Check that the tube is passed to the correct position: mark on tube and listen with stethoscope while small quantity of air is injected. If secretions are produced with pH < 7 = acid, thus tube is in stomach.
6. Attach to drainage bag/pump as instructed and secure appropriately.

7. Make patient comfortable.

8. Management includes aspiration/continuous drainage and accurate measurement and recording of secretions.

9. Give care relating to oral/nasal hygiene.

10. Administer continuous/intermittent feeds.

11. Removal should be carried out swiftly to reduce the risk of vomiting after adequate explanation to the patient.

Peptic ulcer

Key facts

1. An erosion of the mucous membrane which can extend through the muscle layers resulting in perforation.

2. A *perforated* ulcer results in peritonitis, inflammation, paralytic ileus, toxaemia and shock and requires *emergency* surgery.

3. Factors thought to be involved with the development of ulcers include:

(a) familial tendency

(b) poor dietary habits

(c) stress

(d) alcohol intake

(e) smoking.

4. Pain associated with gastric ulcers normally occurs soon after meals and is relieved by vomiting or alkalis.

5. Pain associated with duodenal ulcers often occurs at night or two to three hours after a meal or before the next meal. It is relieved by eating or alkalis.

6. Patients with gastric ulcers will complain of vomiting and weight loss as a result of poor dietary intake.

7. Most patients complain of 'heartburn'.

8. Most ulcers are treated conservatively by general practitioners and/or outpatient departments and *do not* require hospital admission.

9. Surgical procedures include vagotomy, pyloroplasty, gastrectomy.

10. Perforation is normally treated by oversewing.

11. Radical gastrectomy is normally only performed for treatment of carcinoma.

In addition to the above you should ensure you are familiar with the sites of peptic ulceration and the process of gastric secretion, e.g. cephalic, gastric and intestinal phases.

Key aspects of nursing management

1. Directed at relief of the appropriate problems identified above, the assessment and treatment of pain is very important
2. Identification of individual risk factors, e.g emotional stress
3. Promotion of rest and reduction of anxiety
4. Advice to be given to patient on
(a) diet: e.g. avoid curry, seasoning, coffee, alcohol
(b) importance of regular meals
(c) reducing or stopping smoking
(d) avoidance of drugs which cause gastric irritation, e.g. aspirin
(e) medications: antacids, cimetidine
(f) importance of relaxation
(g) appropriate adjustments to lifestyle.

Surgical nursing care should be relevant to the operative procedure and should be based on principles identified in 12.4. (pp. 197–200) and Chapter 7.

You should ensure that you revise the action of commonly used antacids and anti-ulcer drugs, e.g. cimetidine.

Acute appendicitis

Key facts

This is a surgical emergency as rupture will result in peritonitis.

Patients usually complain of pain in the right iliac fossa region, are nauseous and may have vomited. They may also have a slight pyrexia and tachycardia.

For details of specific nursing management you should refer to the worked example in Chapter 7 (pp. 111–14).

Crohn's disease

Key facts

1. It is characterized by inflammation of areas of the alimentary tract separated by normal area.
2. It can occur anywhere in the alimentary tract.
3. Problems experienced by the patient include colicky abdominal pain, diarrhoea, anorexia, weight loss, anaemia, fever if abscess is present.
4. Fistulae can occur between segments of bowel or extend to the skin.
5. There is a familial tendency.
6. There are normally periods of remission and exacerbation.

Key aspects of nursing management
1. Assistance/preparation for medical investigations, e.g. barium meal, enema, abdominal X-rays, rectal examination, collection of blood and stool specimens
2. Administration of prescribed medication and assessment of its effects including specific advice to the patient about steroids, sedatives, vitamin supplements
3. Psychological support and explanations
4. Preparation for surgery appropriate to the site of the lesion – this may initially be resection of a bowel segment but most often a colectomy with formation of an ileostomy is the end result
5. Care of patients with stomas is discussed in 12.5.

Ulcerative colitis

Key facts
1. It is characterized by ulceration and inflammation of the colon and rectum.
2. Problems experienced by the patient include colicky abdominal pain, weight loss, anorexia, anaemia, fever, and diarrhoea which contains mucous and is usually bloodstained.
3. There is a higher incidence in females.
4. The cause is unknown but an autoimmune reaction may be involved.

Key aspects of nursing management
1. Psychological support and counselling about stressful events in the patient's life, and ensuring time is made available to listen and talk to patient
2. Administration of prescribed medication, e.g. anti-inflammatory drugs, steroids
3. Appropriate explanations, support and care relating to investigative procedures, e.g. abdominal X-ray, rectal examinations, sigmoidoscopy and biopsy collection of blood and stool specimens
4. Provision of restful environment and privacy, e.g. side room with adjoining toilet or provision of commode
5. Care relating to problems identified above
6. Observation for and care related to potential complications, e.g. dehydration, tiredness due to anaemia, and excoriation.

Large bowel surgery

Surgery to the large bowel is carried out for a variety of reasons: carcinoma of the colon or rectum are two of the commoner ones. When answering questions relating to care of patients having large bowel surgery it is important to consider what will be the result of the surgery. Many patients *do not* require a colostomy formation and others only require temporary colostomies. It is necessary to take this into account during the preoperative preparation and when planning postoperative care.

Specific preoperative preparation should include:

1. Care relating to relevant preoperative investigations, e.g. rectal examination, sigmoidoscopy
2. Psychological preparation – especially if colostomy formation is planned
3. Physical preparation to achieve the best possible state of health prior to surgery thus reducing the risk of postoperative problems
4. Bowel preparation prior to surgery. This will vary depending on the surgeon's instructions but will *always* be aimed at achieving a sterile bowel, free of faeces, prior to surgery; you should describe the method/régime with which you are familiar in an examination answer
5. Postoperative care must take into account the type of surgery carried out and the health status of the patient prior to surgery.

Specific aspects of postoperative care include:

1. maintenance of fluid/nutritional balance and associated care of intravenous infusion, nasogastric tube, catheter, wound drainage
2. gradual introduction of oral fluids → food after return of bowel sounds
3. mobilization and physiotherapy
4. care relating to colostomy if appropriate (see 12.5. for details)
5. early detection and/or prevention of complications, e.g. wound infection.

12.7. Specific care relating to disorders of other organs

The liver

Key facts

1. Jaundice is a symptom of a problem not an illness.
2. Haemolytic jaundice is due to an abnormally rapid breakdown of red blood cells. There is an excess of unconjugated bilirubin in the blood; no bilirubin is found in the urine but there is an increased urobilinogen level in the urine.

3. Obstructive jaundice can be due to obstruction within the liver itself or externally e.g. gallstones in the common bile duct.

The excess bilirubin in the blood is conjugated and water soluble thus it can be excreted in the urine. Urobilinogen will not be found in the urine as none is being formed in the duodenum because no bilirubin is arriving there due to the obstruction. The stools will be pale or clay-coloured as the normal colour in stools is due to the presence of stercobilinogen which will be absent.

4. Hepatocellular jaundice is due to difficulties in the transport of bilirubin through the hepatic cells. It is commonly due to hepatitis or cirrhosis. Bilirubin is found in the urine but no urobilinogen is present.

5. Cirrhosis is most commonly associated with excessive alcohol consumption and the related nutritional deficiencies. It involves

> destruction of liver cells
> ↓
> scar tissue formation
> ↓
> obstruction of the portal circulation
> ↓
> ascites/varices
> ↓
> chronic liver failure
> ↓
> coma/death.

Ascites are formed as a result of the portal hypertension and the reduced plasma osmotic pressure.

Oesophageal varices are a most serious effect of portal hypertension.

Key aspects of nursing management

In order to plan and deliver effective care to patients suffering from liver disease or problems it is necessary to understand the underlying physiology of liver function in order to anticipate the problems the patient may develop and to provide the most appropriate care for those he already has.

An example of care relating to a patient suffering from liver failure is given in the specimen answer at the end of Chapter 2, with particular reference to gastrointestinal problems.

The following are points which you should always consider when planning care for patients suffering from liver disorders:

1. Is the patient jaundiced? What type of jaundice is it? Is he complaining of pruritis? How severe is it? What nursing action is appropriate? For example

(a) good skin care
(b) no use of soap
(c) use calamine lotion
(d) administer Piriton if prescribed
(e) observe for secondary infection
(f) cut fingernails if patient is scratching.

2. Is oedema present? How severe is it? What nursing action can be taken? For example

(a) Reposition patient regularly, e.g. two-hourly.
(b) Use appropriate aids to relieve pressure.
(c) Maintain accurate fluid balance chart.
(d) Weigh daily.
(e) Elevate extremities.
(f) Administer prescribed medication, e.g. diuretics.

3. Are ascites present? If so, help patient to sit up to facilitate easier breathing. Other care as for 2 above.

   If paracentesis is performed try to ensure patient has bladder/bowel open *before* procedure. Remember to include specific care relating to position, puncture site, dressings, fluids.

4. What gastrointestinal problems are present? For example
anorexia
nausea and vomiting
constipation
diarrhoea
haematemesis
malaena.

   Care relating to these is identified in the sample answer on pp. 29–33.

5. Is he in pain? To what degree? Where is it? What type is it?
   Pain can be relieved by:

(a) ensuring bed rest to rest liver
(b) maintaining comfortable position in bed including frequent changes of position
(c) administration of prescribed anti-spasmodics; analgesics. N.B. Remember, strong analgesics would not be effectively metabolized in liver failure.

6. What is his mental state – lethargic, depressed, confused, stuporous, comatose?

   Give appropriate psychological support and care.

7. Are there haemorrhagic problems? What?

Nursing action includes care relating to mouth and gums, e.g. do not use a toothbrush; avoid trauma to patient; use small-bore needles; advise patient to avoid bruising.

8. What other care is required?

Care appropriate to the specific stage in his illness, e.g. acute failure; terminal care.

You are unlikely to be asked to discuss acute management of severely bleeding oesophageal varices but remember this is an emergency requiring resuscitation or the patient will die due to massive blood loss. Care is thus directed at: restoring haemodynamic status; assisting medical staff with treatment, e.g. insertion of central venous line – Swan-Ganz catheter; insertion of Sengstaken or Minnesota tube.

Remember that as part of a longer question you could be asked to discuss factors associated with liver failure or cirrhosis, e.g. excessive alcohol intake and relate this to social factors or health education work (see Chapter 4).

Care of patients with hepatitis is discussed in Chapter 17.

The gall bladder

Key facts

1. Its function is to store and concentrate bile.
2. It is not essential to life.
3. The presence of fat in the duodenum causes the release of cholecystokinin (C.C.K.) into the blood circulation. C.C.K. then stimulates the gall bladder to contract.
4. Cholecystitis is inflammation of the gall bladder and the patient normally complains of acute pain and tenderness in the upper abdominal region and associated dyspepsia, nausea and vomiting, especially following meals containing fatty foods. It can be caused by gallstones and, more frequently, infection.
5. Most gallstones (cholelithiasis) are composed predominantly of cholesterol. If obstruction of the bile ducts by gallstones occurs the patient may, in addition to the above points, complain of intense pain referred to the right shoulder, fever and associated sweating and rigors.

Key aspects of nursing management

1. Observation of urine and faeces for evidence of obstructive jaundice
2. Assistance with preparation for oral cholecystogram: fasting overnight after taking, for example, Telepaque tablets; X-rays are taken the next

morning followed by a fatty meal and further X-rays to see if the gall bladder contracts (an intravenous cholangiogram is carried out by administering the radio-opaque dye in the X-ray department approximately ten minutes prior to taking the X-rays).

3. *Preoperatively*:

(a) The nurse should ensure that appropriate medical results are available, e.g. X-ray results, blood test results, i.e. liver function tests, haemoglobin level.

(b) Explain operation and postoperative care, e.g. drainage tubes, pain relief, position in bed.

(c) Administer prescribed medications, e.g. vitamin K if prothrombin level is low; intramuscular analgesia for pain relief.

(d) Routine preoperative preparation (see Chapter 7).

4. *Postoperatively*: routine care as in Chapter 7.

Specifically:

(a) Aspirate nasogastric tube to relieve nausea.

(b) Sit upright and well supported to facilitate easier breathing once recovered from effects of anaesthetic.

(c) Encourage deep breathing.

(d) Teach to support wound when coughing.

(e) Management of intravenous infusion until bowel sounds return and oral fluids/diet tolerated.

(f) Care of drainage from gall bladder bed, e.g. via Yates drain; measurement of drainage, shortening and removal of drain after forty-eight hours as instructed.

(g) Care of T tube if used (e.g. following exploration of the common bile duct), measure and record drainage; clamp tube as instructed; following T tube cholangiogram, after approximately seven days remove tube as instructed ensuring prescribed analgesia is administered first.

(h) Observation of wound, drain site, T tube site for leakage of bile.

(i) Accurate assessment of fluid balance.

(j) Observation of urine and stools for evidence of bile pigments.

(k) Encourage return to normal diet.

(l) Referral to dietitian for dietary advice, e.g. related to losing weight if obese; restriction of fats for approximately four weeks until bile ducts have dilated to accommodate increased bile flow.

12.8. Specimen R.G.N. questions

Q.1. Mrs Jessie Phillips, a 60-year-old housewife in the terminal stages of abdominal carcinoma, has been readmitted to hospital for treatment of severe ascites. Her husband is retired and, until now, has cared for her adequately. They have no children.

With specific reference to the causes of her pain and discomfort, give an account of Mrs Phillips's nursing care and management prior to her return home. 100%

Final R.G.N. paper, English and Welsh National Board, March 1985

Q.2. Mrs Joanne Kershaw is an obese, 40-year-old mother of 3-year-old twins. She has a part-time job in a school canteen and her husband is a regular night worker. Mrs Kershaw has undergone a cholecystectomy and exploration of the common bile duct and is conscious on her return to the ward from the operating theatre.

(a) Describe the postoperative care that Mrs Kershaw will require until her discharge. 65%

(b) Identify the problems Mrs Kershaw may encounter following her discharge home and discuss how these may be resolved. 35%

Final R.G.N. paper, English and Welsh National Board, March 1985

Q.3. Mrs Enid Andrews, aged 43 years, is married and has a 12-year-old daughter. She is admitted at 02.00 hours with acute intestinal obstruction, thought to be due to adhesions following a previous appendicectomy.

(a) Describe the nursing measures likely to be taken until Mrs Andrews goes to the operating theatre. 60%

(b) Describe the nursing care Mrs Andrews will require during the first six months after her operation. 40%

Final R.G.N. paper, English and Welsh National Board, July 1984

12.9. Sample question and answer

Q. Mrs Velda Raymond, a 53-year-old nurse, who lives with her husband and 20-year-old daughter, has been admitted to the ward following an emergency resection of the colon for a perforated diverticulum.

(a) Describe the nursing care and management Mrs Raymond will require *following her return to the ward until her discharge*   70%

(*b*) *What advice would Mrs Raymond be given on discharge to help prevent further episodes of diverticulitis?*   30%

(*a*) Key points to include are:

initial care

observations

early mobilization

psychological support

involvement of family

general care.

Remember she has had a *resection* of the colon *not* formation of a colostomy although sometimes this may be formed temporarily.

1. *Initial care*:

(a) Position in bed to maintain airway.

(b) Observe for signs of shock/infection.

(c) Make frequent assessment initially of vital signs.

(d) Observe wound, drainage tubes.

(e) Aspirate or continuously drain nasogastric tube.

(f) Maintain intravenous infusion.

(g) Administer pain relief.

(h) Give nil fluids orally.

(i) Note time and amount of urine passed and observe for evidence of retention.

2. *After initial period*:

(a) Position appropriately in bed in relation to haemodynamic status.

(b) Give face and hands wash and provide clean nightdress.

(c) Help to change position to relieve pressure.

(d) Maintain accurate fluid balance chart.

(e) Continue observations as in 1 but reduce frequency.

(f) Encourage leg/chest physiotherapy.

(g) Help her to sit out of bed on first day postoperatively.

(h) Assist patient in maintenance of basic hygiene needs, e.g. by giving bed bath, mouthwashes.

(i) Withhold oral fluids until bowel sounds return and then commence with gradually increasing amounts.

(j) Remove naso-gastric tube when fluids are being absorbed adequately.

(k) Discontinue intravenous infusion when adequate oral fluid intake.

(l) Commence diet slowly when fluids tolerated.

(m) Encourage mobility towards independence.

(n) Allow patient to take increased responsibility for her basic care/satisfaction of needs.

(o) Continue to carry out appropriate wound care, e.g. remove drains; remove sutures after seven to ten days; observe for evidence of infection.

(p) Encourage fluids and exercise.

(q) Prevent constipation.

3. *Psychological support*:

(a) Explain about operation.

(b) Reassure her that she has not got cancer.

(c) Encourage independence.

(d) Promote positive attitude to work, family, returning home.

(e) Involve family in above points.

(f) Relate to her own knowledge and nursing experience as appropriate.

(*b*)

1. Explain about diverticulitis; build on her knowledge.

2. Stress should be laid on the importance of reporting early signs of recurrence to her general practitioner, e.g. low-grade fever, bowel irregularity, abdominal pain.

3. Advise her of the importance of avoiding constipation and ensuring regular bowel actions, she should use laxatives if necessary and avoid straining. Give her advice on diet and fibre intake; fluid intake.

4. Regular exercise should be taken.

5. Regular, for example, three-monthly, check-ups at outpatient department.

N.B. It is important to remember that she is a nurse and to take this into account when giving your advice.

Examples of other questions with sample answers relating to abdominal problems can be found at the ends of Chapters 2 and 7.

13. Care of patients with orthopaedic problems

13.1. Fractures

A fracture is a break in the continuity of bone.

Types of fracture

The following terms may be used to describe a fracture:
Complete: across entire cross-section of the bone
Incomplete: across part of the cross-section of the bone
Open (compound): extends through the skin
Closed (simple): does not communicate with the outside area.
(a) Transverse: straight across the bone
(b) Comminuted: involves the bone splitting
(c) Greenstick: one side of the bone is broken while the other is bent
(d) Impacted: the broken bone is wedged into another bone
(e) Spiral: involves twisting around the shaft of the bone.
    It is very important to know exactly what these terms mean as the care and treatment of each patient is different depending on the type of fracture.

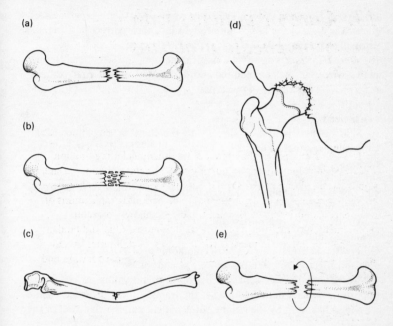

(a)

(b)

(c)

(d)

(e)

The healing process for fractures

This starts off with the formation of a haematoma, which leads on to a granulation process and the formation of a connective tissue/cartilage bridge across the fracture. This bridge is called callus. Calcium is then deposited which causes ossification. The final hardening process, over many weeks, is called consolidation.

Osteoblasts are bone-forming cells responsible for new bone.

Osteoclasts are bone-destroying cells responsible for shaping the bone.

Treatment of fractures

The principles are always the same:
1. reduction
2. immobilization
3. rehabilitation.
1. Reduction means restoring the bones to their normal anatomical position. There are three ways in which this is achieved.

(a) *Closed reduction* is done manually, normally under a general anaesthetic; the ends of the bones are brought into their correct position and normally a plaster of Paris cast is applied.

(b) *Open reduction* is done via a surgical incision, and screws, nails, pins, plates, wires, etc, may be required in order to carry out internal fixation.

(c) *Traction*: this can be of two types:

(i) skin

(ii) skeletal.

(i) Skin traction is applied directly to the skin via a commercial kit containing Elastoplast or foam extension which is bandaged to hold it in place.

(ii) Skeletal traction is applied directly to a bone. Usually a metal pin, e.g. Denham or Steinman, is driven through the bone to form a point of attachment for the traction.

Skin traction is appropriate for children or for immobilization prior to surgery and postoperatively for elderly patients with hip fractures. Otherwise, skeletal traction is most commonly used as it is more comfortable and effective and suitable for long periods of use.

Most traction is *balanced*. This is done by providing an equal and opposite counter traction force; i.e. the traction force provided by the weights is balanced by the weight of the patient and the elevation of the foot of the bed.

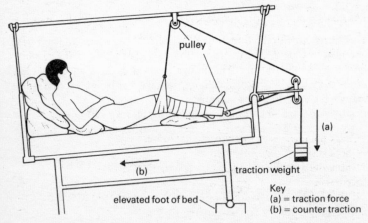

Key
(a) = traction force
(b) = counter traction

2. Immobilization is the way in which the bones are held in position after reduction so as to allow the fracture to heal. This may be in plaster of Paris, by use of splints or slings, or by other appropriate measures.

3. Rehabilitation means the restoration of the full use of the limb and is an ongoing process which starts as soon as the patient returns from theatre. It includes exercises and movement within the limitations of the form of immobilization.

General points to be considered when preparing to admit an orthopaedic patient
1. Have the correct type of bed, i.e. firm mattress, backrest, can be raised and lowered, and ensure that any traction required will fit into it.
2. Make sure it is in an appropriate position for the patient's condition and the safety of other patients and staff.
3. Collect any extra equipment which may be required for traction and/or immobilization in advance.
4. Ensure adequate pillows and bedcradle are available.

13.2. Specific observations on nursing care

Skeletal traction

The following points must be included when caring for patients with skeletal traction:
1. Ensure correct weights are applied and do not readjust them or lift them off.
2. Ensure weights are hanging freely and not resting on the bed or floor.
3. Check the cord is running freely over the pulleys.
4. Ensure the system is balanced, i.e. that counter traction is applied.
5. Make sure knots in the cords are secure.
6. Ensure limb is correctly aligned.

Pin site

1. Check pin is correctly in place and not loose.
2. Check stirrup is correctly fitted.
3. Check site for signs of oozing or inflammation.
4. Redress aseptically as appropriate.
5. If there is a discharge present, take specimen and send to laboratory for microscopy, culture and sensitivity.

Skin traction

1. Observe limb for condition of skin, i.e. do not use if sensory loss, eczema, ulcers.
2. Observe limb for signs of oedema.
3. Do not bandage too tightly and apply bandage evenly, i.e. figure-of-eight style.
4. Allow a gap between the heel and the end of the skin extensions to prevent sores and allow movement and exercises.
5. Rebandage at least twice a day if foam extensions are used.
6. Always bandage from the heel upwards.
7. Wash limb when rebandaging as patient often finds skin traction irritating and causing him to sweat.
8. Ensure correct weights are applied.

Plaster of Paris

1. *Initially*:
(a) Elevate on pillows or Braun frame.
(b) Use plastic drawsheet to protect bed from wet plaster.
(c) Use palms of hands not fingers to support limb.
(d) Do not cover limb with blankets but allow to dry by evaporation.
(e) Examine plaster for cracks and weakness.
(f) Observe plaster for signs of oozing from wound and mark with biro; regularly reassess.
(g) Check limb for colour, temperature, sensation, movement, numbness and tingling.
(h) Report persistent pain or swelling to doctor.
(i) Explain to patient that heat is generated from the plaster while it is drying but that it will cool down when dry.
2. *Long term*:
(a) Cut window in plaster to carry out aseptic dressings to wound site if appropriate.
(b) Ensure plaster does not get wet when washing patient or when he is using bedpan.
(c) Examine plaster as above.
(d) Ensure limb is correctly supported when it has dried.
   In your answer to an examination question always say where plaster cast is from and to, and whether there is flexion incorporated in it, e.g. toes to groin with foot held in dorsiflexion.
   Remember, most plaster casts suitable for prolonged immobilization

may not be suitable for walking on. Therefore, they will need changing before the patient can weightbear.

13.3. First aid measures; care in accident and emergency departments

When answering questions related especially to compound fractures you may be asked to describe first aid measures taken at the scene or in the accident and emergency department. Also, remember that *total* care of a patient in hospital includes care in the accident and emergency department.

First aid measures should include:
1. Summoning help, ambulance
2. Not moving patient unnecessarily
3. Splinting the limb *before* movement: supporting it above and below the fracture site, by using, for example, bandages, padding, strapping the legs together, etc.

If the fracture is compound, cover the wound with a clean piece of material and try to reduce haemorrhage by applying pressure around the wound site. Do not press directly on to protruding bone fragments.

Measures taken in the accident and emergency departments

These should include:
1. assessing the patient for other injuries and keeping the limb immobilized
2. carrying out observations of temperature, pulse, blood pressure, respirations (and conscious level if appropriate)
3. obtaining a history of the accident from the patient or relative
4. giving analgesia as prescribed
5. giving tetanus toxoid and antibiotics as prescribed if it is a compound fracture
6. finding out when patient last had a meal and ensuring they remain 'nil orally'
7. assisting the doctor with X-rays, examination, blood tests and care of intravenous infusion
8. removing clothes and general preparation for theatre
9. explaining everything to the patient and supporting the relatives or informing them if they do not know of the patient's admission

10. if it is a compound fracture then careful wound toilet may be carried out
11. inform the ward of the patient's admission and arrange transfer.

13.4. *Serious complications of orthopaedic injuries*

1. For compound fractures the risk of infection is of paramount importance, i.e. tetanus, osteomyelitis and gas gangrene.

Gas gangrene is due to Gram positive Clostridia and as these bacteria do not require oxygen to survive (anaerobic) they thrive in deep wounds. They are resistant to treatment once infection has set in, except hyperbaric oxygen therapy, and can rapidly cause death. Foul, frothy liquid is produced from the wound and gas 'crackles' in the tissues.

Osteomyelitis and tetanus are preventable if tetanus toxoid is given in the accident and emergency department and, if appropriate, antibiotics are provided and given to the patient to prevent other infections.

2. *Hypovolaemic shock* may occur due to haemorrhage into the tissues especially following a fracture to the femur or the pelvis.

3. *Fat embolism* due to fat globules being released from the yellow bone marrow into the bloodstream and lodging in, for example, branches of the pulmonary artery, causing severe chest pain, increased respirations and dyspnoea, can be fatal if not detected early and treated.

13.5. *Specific fractures*

The following sections list points to remember about specific types of fracture.

Fractures in children

General points
As children's bones are softer they tolerate some degree of 'bending' and thus do not fracture as easily as those of adults. They are, however, most likely to suffer greenstick fractures.

As their bones are still growing and have a good blood supply they are likely to heal more quickly, though damage to the epiphysis may affect growth and for this reason skeletal traction is rarely applied to children.

Two important examples of fractures in children are:
1. Supracondylar fracture of the humerus, which carries, in nursing

care, the risk of irritation or injury to the brachial artery, thus causing Volkman's ischaemic contracture. Children with this type of fracture are always kept in hospital for approximately forty-eight hours and closely observed.

Specific observations include:

(a) the radial pulse on the affected side
(b) the colour, warmth and sensation of the fingers
(c) pain in the forearm, especially when extending the fingers
(d) constriction due to the bandage or plaster of Paris
(e) compression due to oedema or increased flexion

2. Fracture of the shaft of the femur. In young children this is treated by using gallows traction:

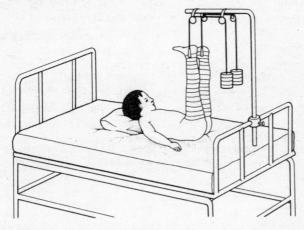

Specific points to include in an answer are:

(a) care to be taken in correct application of the skin traction and weights
(b) ensuring buttocks do not rest on the bed
(c) regular skin care
(d) checking circulation in limb
(e) help with feeding and hygiene difficulties.

In older children the treatment can be by fixed traction. This normally consists of skin traction tied to the end of a Thomas splint to reduce and then immobilize the limb.

Total hip replacement (arthroplasty)

Patients are normally elderly and have suffered from osteoarthritis for a long time causing them both pain and deformity. Conservative measures such as analgesia, physiotherapy and various aids to walking will have been tried first.

Two major procedures are used:
1. Replacing the head of the femur with a prosthesis, e.g. Moore's or Thompson's. This involves implanting the prosthesis into the shaft of the femur and either fixing with cement (Thompson's) or allowing bone consolidation to take place through holes in the metal prosthesis (Moore's).
2. Replacing the hip joint, e.g. McKee-Farrar or Charnley. McKee-Farrar involves using a studded acetabular cup in addition to a modified Thompson's prosthesis. Charnley involves using a plastic acetabular cup and a small metal femoral head.

The choice of treatment depends on the type of fracture and the surgeon's preference. There are other types of prosthesis used and you should consult your teachers and ward sister for details of these if they are used in your hospital.

Preoperative nursing care

1. These patients are often elderly, therefore the nurse should anticipate potential postoperative problems by a good initial nursing assessment.
For example,
What is the patient's skin condition like?
How mobile is he?
Has he a urinary or chest infection?
Is he underweight or in a poor nutritional state?
2. Try to teach the patient quadriceps muscle exercises, how to use crutches and to non-weightbear on the affected side if at all possible as it will help with postoperative recovery.
3. Explain what an abduction pillow is and how and why it is used as well as why skin traction may be used.
4. All basic preoperative preparation would be carried out as normal (Chapter 7) but important points to remember are skin cleaning; full-length shave of the leg; iodine patch test; ensuring chest X-ray, electro-cardiograph (E.C.G.), and full blood count and cross-match have been carried out.
5. Leg immobilized with skin traction and placed in a 'gutter splint'.

Postoperative nursing care

1. The patient should normally lie flat initially, but be raised to semi-recumbent position by approximately twenty-four hours.

2. The legs are maintained in an abducted position and the patient should not be turned on to his side until the doctor has arranged an X-ray of the joint and is satisfied it is stable.

3. Patients who have had a posterior approach may have to remain flat or semi-recumbent for approximately one week.

4. When turning the patient ensure the hip is kept abducted and the leg supported with pillows.

5. Avoid flexion and adduction when using a bedpan.

6. In addition to normal postoperative care (see Chapter 7) check and compare the colour, temperature and pulses of the leg with the unoperated side.

7. Correctly maintain the skin traction if used.

8. The Redivac drain is normally removed after forty-eight hours.

9. Exercises are commenced on the first day. Give analgesia before the physiotherapist arrives and the patient (unless a posterior approach) should be able to get up to use a commode on the third day.

10. The patient should be flat for an hour at least once a day to prevent flexion contractures.

11. Sutures are normally removed after ten to fourteen days and by then the patient should be mobile with crutches or a tripod.

12. Advise the patient of the types of movement to avoid on discharge, e.g. crossing legs, twisting excessively. Also, ensure he understands how to use his stick, crutches or tripod. Make arrangements for physiotherapy and outpatient appointments.

When answering a question about care of this type of patient remember to direct your care to avoiding *adduction*, *forced flexion* and *external rotation* as all these movements may cause dislocation. Also, as these patients are elderly they are very susceptible to deep vein thromboses, pulmonary embolism, pressure sores, infection and dehydration and this must be taken into account when discussing their care.

Hip fractures

Mostly seen in elderly people. They involve the head, neck or trochanter of the femur. They are treated by a 'pin and plate' procedure whereby nails and a metal plate are used to fix the position of the bone fragments. If this is not possible then a total hip replacement is performed.

Preoperative care is similar to that following a total hip replacement.

Postoperatively the patient should be able to be out of bed and walking with a frame after a few days. He will remain non-weightbearing on the affected limb until the surgeon is satisfied that sufficient bone healing has taken place. There is no risk of postoperative dislocation as with total hip replacement and the early mobilization decreases the chance of complications of bed rest.

Potts fracture

This is a fracture dislocation of the ankle joint involving the lower end of the tibia and fibula.

The treatment is reduction via manipulation followed by application of a plaster cast with the foot held in a right-angled position. The plaster cast is applied from the toes to just below the knee.

Postoperatively the patient is nursed in bed with the leg elevated on pillows. If the fracture is stable he can get up weightbearing after a few days. If not, he will remain on bed rest or up in a wheelchair with the leg elevated until the fracture is stable, when an unpadded plaster cast will be applied and he will be able to weightbear.

Windows will normally be cut in the plaster casts to carry out aseptic dressings as these fractures are usually compound.

Other ankle/tendon injuries also require plaster casts for six to twelve weeks.

Fracture of tibia and fibula (*shaft*)

Treatment is normally reduction by manipulation followed by immobilization in a plaster cast. The plaster cast is usually made so that there is approximately 15 degrees flexion at the knee, and the plaster extends from the toes up to the groin.

If the fracture is unstable after reduction, skeletal traction may be used. A Denham pin is then put through the os calcis or the lower end of the shaft of the femur and this is incorporated within the plaster cast.

Postoperative care
1. The bed is elevated and the leg elevated on pillows or a Braun frame.
2. All the standard observations made on patients with plaster casts (see 13.2) should also be included in your answer.
3. This is almost always a compound fracture therefore observations for early detection of infection must be included: i.e. regular (four-hourly) recording of temperature or pulse; aseptic dressings to wound via windows

in plaster; send swabs for microscopy, culture and sensitivity if infection suspected; give prescribed antibiotics.

The length of time on bed rest depends on the rate of healing of the fracture but may be between six and fourteen weeks. When there is evidence on X-rays of callus formation the plaster can be changed to a weightbearing one and the patient can begin to walk again.

Fractured femur (shaft)

In adults, the action of the powerful leg muscles causes shortening and rotation of the limb so this cannot be treated by skin traction. If the fracture is just below the trochanter, it may be treated with open reduction and internal fixation with a Küntscher nail. The patient can then be up non-weightbearing with crutches in approximately three weeks.

If the fracture is in the mid-shaft then continuous skeletal traction is necessary. Balanced suspended (or sliding) traction is used. The limb is immobilized in a well-padded Thomas splint. Continuous traction is applied via a pin through the upper tibia. This is balanced by the effect of the patient's weight and elevating the end of the bed. The immobilized limb is suspended via pulleys so that the limb and the patient's body are able to move in the bed as a single unit.

The patient is likely to spend at least twelve weeks in bed and will not be fully weightbearing for approximately six months.

When answering questions relating to postoperative care it is important to include observations relating to the skeletal traction and the pin site (see 13.2) as well as general postoperative observations.

Patients with fractures of the femur and tibia and fibula are usually young and often male. It is therefore very important to consider the social and psychological effects of long-term bed rest as well as the physical care in your answer. For example, the effect on marriage or other relationships; possible loss of job; which benefits are available; anxiety over insurance or court appearances; boredom and frustration.

Knee injuries

Most commonly, a rotation injury involving the tearing of the medial meniscus. The treatment is removal of the meniscus by a meniscectomy.

Specific preoperative care
1. Intensive quadriceps muscle exercises
2. Skin preparation from toes to groin.

Specific postoperative care
1. Robert Jones bandage applied directly over the knee
2. Splinting of limb in full extension to metal backsplint
3. Quadriceps exercises for five minutes every hour
4. If the patient is young, then allow up in a wheelchair with leg elevated after a few days. Removal of sutures and splint after eight to ten days. If quadriceps is strong and knee controlled, the patient may then be up weightbearing.

A Robert Jones bandage is a pressure bandage consisting of a layer of splint wool followed by three fine turns of crepe bandage, followed by another layer of splint wool and three more turns of bandage.

Pelvic fractures

Most patients with pelvic fractures have other injuries as well. They are normally treated by bed rest with gentle movement for about six weeks by which time they have healed sufficiently for the patient to weightbear.

Such injuries are serious, however, because of risk of haemorrhage into the retroperitoneal region and danger of laceration to veins, arteries, bladder, urethra and intestine from bone fragments.

Specific nursing observations
1. Signs of shock: ↑pulse, ↓blood pressure, sweating, pallor
2. Signs of urinary tract damage: passing blood in urine; unable to pass urine; pain on micturition
3. Checking of abdominal girth for increase indicating haemorrhage
4. Checking of limb pulses in case of damage to iliac artery.

Back injuries

A prolapsed intervertebral disc occurs when the central nucleus pulposus herniates into the posterior part of the annulus.

Initial treatment consists of analgesia, muscle relaxants and anti-inflammatory drugs in addition to bed rest. Manipulation, corsets and traction may also be tried. If these fail then surgery to remove the nucleus pulposus is performed. This is called a *laminectomy*.

Specific preoperative care
1. Low-residue diet
2. Iodine patch test
3. Skin preparation.

Specific postoperative care
1. At least one week should be spent flat, on bed rest.
2. Allow one pillow under head.
3. Use bedcradle.
4. Encourage slight knee flexion.
5. Check limbs for colour, temperature, motor power and sensation.
6. Observe for urinary retention.
7. Turn two-hourly by 'log-rolling', pillow between legs and without twisting the back.
8. When sitting up gradually keep knees flexed.
9. Weightbearing after two to four weeks.
10. Wear a corset for approximately three months.
11. When up, the patient should still lie flat in bed for at least one hour twice a day.
12. Sutures are usually removed after two weeks.
13. Emphasis must be placed on caring for the patient's eating, drinking and elimination needs.
14. Educate about exercises, rest and avoiding heavy work for at least three months after discharge.

If extensive spinal fusion is performed as well then the patient may be nursed on a specially made plaster bed for up to three months and then have a plaster jacket for a further one to two months.

Spinal injuries

The care these patients require depends on two important factors:
1. The level of the lesion
2. Whether the cord is completely transected or not.

If the lesion is above the fourth neurological cervical segment then the patient will be paralysed in all four limbs – *tetraplegia* – and will have respiratory problems.

If the lesion is below the eighth neurological cervical segment then the patient will be able to use the arms and only be paralysed in the legs – *paraplegia*.

If the lesion is complete then no nerve impulses pass down the cord below the level of transection. If it is incomplete then some nerve fibres will still allow impulses through causing a variety of symptoms especially muscle spasm in the lower limbs.

Acute care

1. Keep patient flat and immobile.
2. Never bend the neck or back.
3. Nurse patient on a turning frame such as the Stryker frame or an electric bed, such as the Stoke Mandeville bed. Turn patient using either of these two-hourly (or lift the patient two-hourly ensuring the head, neck and spine remain in a straight line to prevent further injury).
4. Carry out all basic needs for patient.

Long-term care

1. *Psychological.* Patient goes through stages often over many months before acceptance, i.e. shock → denial → depression → acceptance.

As patients are often young relate your answer to their social situation, employment, future prospects and potential after full rehabilitation.

Never do too much for the patient and always allow them time to complete tasks like dressing.

2. *Physical.*

(a) Turning patient two-hourly is vital as pressure sores occur very quickly in paralysed limbs. They also heal very slowly because of poor circulation and muscle wasting. The patients cannot turn themselves and have often lost sensation in the affected limbs and thus cannot feel themselves getting sore.

(b) Careful positioning of limbs with pillows is vital. Use a bedcradle to relieve pressure. Ensure sheets and pyjamas are not wrinkled.

(c) Carry out passive limb movements each time the patient is turned. Do not leave the limbs in spasm. (Spasm means involuntary contraction of the muscle groups, seen in patients with incomplete lesions.) Ensure the foot is properly positioned and supported.

(d) The patient will have lost bowel control so establish a regular routine using aperients, suppositories and/or manual evacuation. Do not use bedpans other than rubber ones because of the risk of damaging the skin. Ensure good fluid intake and diet.

(e) Bladder control will have been lost so if possible try to establish a routine by using manual pressure if no reflex activity is present. Use aids such as condoms and drainage bags where possible and a catheter only as a last resort because of the risk of infection.

Rehabilitation is a long process and is best achieved in specialist spinal injury centres.

13.6. Specimen R.G.N. question

Q. Miss Howard, a 65-year-old retired school-teacher who lives with her elderly sister, has osteoarthritis of the right hip. She is admitted to hospital for hip replacement.

Using a problem-solving approach, describe Miss Howard's postoperative management until the time of her discharge from hospital. 100%

Final R.G.N. paper, English and Welsh National Board, March 1984

13.7. Sample question and answer

Q. John Watson, an 18-year-old student, is admitted to the accident and emergency department following a motorcycle accident. He has sustained a fracture to the shaft of his right femur.

(a) What nursing care should John receive in the accident and emergency department? 30%

(b) Describe John's care during the twenty-four hours following his admission to the ward. 70%

(a) Answer plan

1. Observations of vital signs – pulse, respirations, blood pressure, conscious level. Record and report significant changes which may be due to shock and haemorrhage.

2. Examine for other injuries.

3. Assist with X-rays, medical examination and treatment, e.g. setting up of intravenous infusion or blood transfusion.

4. Give analgesia as prescribed.

5. Removal of clothes, record property and valuables and deal with them appropriately.

6. Give nil orally and check when John last ate.

7. Explain all procedures to John and ensure his consent has been obtained prior to surgery.

8. Carry out safety and identification checks prior to surgery.

9. Contact relatives and reassure John that this has been done. Do not leave him alone.

10. Inform the ward of his admission and arrange for his transfer to the ward after theatre.

(*b*)

General care

1. Maintenance of airway.

2. Care of blood transfusion or intravenous infusion.

3. Observe and record vital signs – pulse, respirations, blood pressure, half-hourly. Then hourly until stable, then four-hourly.

4. Report any significant changes, e.g. indicating shock.

5. Check colour of right leg and toes.

6. Observe for signs of deep vein thrombosis: swelling, pain, and heat in calf.

7. Observe for signs of pulmonary/fat embolus: increased respiration, dyspnoea, cough and chest pain.

8. Give appropriate analgesia: intramuscularly, e.g. Omnopon, 20 mg as prescribed.

9. Ensure John is comfortable, positioned on his back with pillows to support his head.

10. Give postoperative wash and clean pyjamas when awake. Give mouthwashes until he is able to tolerate fluids.

11. Observe John's pressure areas and lift two-hourly to avoid soreness to sacral area. Encourage John to use a 'monkey pole' when able. Check sheets for creases or crumbs.

12. Give help with daily hygiene needs but encourage independence.

13. Provide urinal for use. Ensure privacy.

14. Encourage fluids and high protein, high carbohydrate diet.

15. Explain to John about his treatment and care.

16. Involve family as far as possible.

Specific care

1. Care of traction: state clearly what is used. For example, skeletal traction, e.g. Denham pin through upper tibia; limb immobilized in Thomas splint; pulleys and weights as requested by doctor.

2. Check that weights are hanging freely and are secure and that the cords are firmly fixed and of adequate length.

3. Check that the whole system runs smoothly over the pulley and all fixing points, that the stirrup attached to the Denham pin is secure.

4. Ensure the Thomas splint is the correct size and fitting.

5. Check pin site for oozing and re-dress aseptically.

13.8. Multiple choice questions

Q.1. Which one of these statements describes the nursing priority *following a total hip replacement?*
(a) *prevention of abduction of hip*
(b) *turning patient on to the unaffected side*
(c) *prevention of adduction of hip*
(d) *turning the patient on to the affected side.*

The correct answer is (c) because the movement of adduction (crossing the legs by moving the affected limb towards the midline over the body) is likely to result in dislocation.

(a) is wrong because you should be maintaining the hip in a position of abduction. (b) and (d) are wrong because they reflect the policy of the doctor and will thus vary depending on where you work.

Q.2. A man with skeletal traction in situ for a fractured shaft of femur complains he is slipping down the bed frequently. Which one of the following is the most likely reason for this?
(a) *He does not have enough pillows.*
(b) *He has too many weights on his traction.*
(c) *He is not being nursed on a sheepskin.*
(d) *Counter traction is not being applied.*

(d) is the correct answer because this will balance the effect of the pull from the traction weights, thus elevate the bed.

(a) and (c) are wrong because neither will prevent nor encourage him to slip down the bed. (b) is wrong because it is unlikely the weights could pull him down the bed if it is elevated and they are correctly applied.

Q.3. Which one of the following is the first stage in the healing of fractures?
(a) *callus formation*
(b) *haematoma formation*
(c) *osteoblast activity*
(d) *deposition of mineral salts.*

(b) is the correct answer because this is bound to occur where bleeding is taking place.

(a) is wrong because callus is formed after (b). (c) is wrong because it refers to bone-forming cells which cannot affect the healing process until after (b) has taken place. (d) does not occur until (a) has formed.

Q.4. Which one of the following statements implies that internal fixation has taken place?
(*a*) *The joint is immovable.*
(*b*) *An open reduction was done.*
(*c*) *A plaster cast is* in situ.
(*d*) *Skeletal traction is in use.*

(*b*) is the correct answer as internal fixation can only occur if an open reduction is performed (that is, via a wound or incision in the skin).

(*a*) may or may not be true but cannot be implied from the statement. (*c*) is likely to follow internal fixation but can apply to many other situations as well. (*d*) skeletal traction can be in use for many other reasons and thus this answer is wrong.

14. Care of patients with genitourinary problems

14.1. Introduction 14.2. Key facts relating to relevant anatomy and physiology 14.3. Care of patients with genitourinary tract infections: cystitis; pyelonephritis 14.4. Specific care relating to patients having major surgery: renal; prostatic 14.5. Care relating to other renal problems: acute renal failure: chronic renal failure: nephrotic syndrome: acute glomerulonephritis; chronic glomerulonephritis 14.6. Specimen R.G.N. questions 14.7. Sample question and answer 14.8. Multiple choice questions

14.1. Introduction

This chapter includes some key facts relating to relevant anatomy and physiology but students should refer to their textbooks and lecture notes for the greater depth of information which they will be expected to have.

Relevant tests and investigations are mentioned at appropriate points. The topics covered in this chapter reflect the major conditions that the student should be familiar with and include those topics most likely to be asked about in a final R.G.N. examination paper.

Gynaecological topics are covered separately in Chapter 15.

14.2. Key facts relating to anatomy and physiology

N.B. You would be expected to be familiar with the gross and microscopic structure of the kidney.

Functions of the *kidney* are:
1. Excretion of waste products and formation of urine
2. Water and electrolyte balance
3. Production of erythropoietin
4. Maintenance of blood pH.

It is also involved in blood-volume regulation via the renin-angiotensin system and calcium metabolism through vitamin D conversion.

Only molecules of molecular weight <68,000 can be filtered at the glomerulus, e.g. H_2O; glucose; amino acids; urea; creatinine. Molecules of molecular weight >68,000 cannot be filtered, e.g. plasma proteins, platelets, red and white blood cells.

Glucose and amino acids are normally completely reabsorbed in the proximal convoluted tubule as is 80 per cent of the H_2O.

Approximately 120 cm^3 fluid is filtered per minute at the glomerulus (170 litres per day); 99 per cent is reabsorbed. Thus normally 1½ litres of urine are produced daily on average.

H_2O reabsorption in the collecting ducts is under the control of the anti-diuretic hormone (A.D.H.) which is secreted from the *neurohypophysis* and renders the cells of the walls of the collecting duct permeable to H_2O. When there is *no* circulating A.D.H. the walls of the collecting duct are virtually impermeable to H_2O.

The ability of the kidney to concentrate solutes is shown by measurements of specific gravity and osmolality. The rate of glomerular filtration is indicated by the *clearance* of a substance. Creatinine is commonly used as the amount filtered at the glomerulus is approximately equal to the amount excreted. It is calculated from:

$$\text{Clearance of C} = \frac{\text{urine volume per unit of time} \times \text{urine concentration of C}}{\text{plasma concentration of C}}$$

which requires the collection of urine over twenty-four hours and the taking of blood specimens.

14.3. *Care of patients with genitourinary tract infections*

Cystitis

Factors contributing to infection in women
1. Short female urethra
2. Close proximity of urethral orifice to vagina and anus
3. Reflux of urine from the urethra into the bladder
4. Stasis of urine in the bladder
5. Utero-vaginal displacement
6. Urinary tract obstruction
7. Catheterization; cystoscopy; trauma to urethral mucosa
8. Faecal contamination
9. May be associated with sexual intercourse.

N.B. Men are much less likely to develop cystitis as they have a longer urethra and their prostate secretions have antibacterial properties.

The patient usually complains of frequency, urgency, nocturia, strangury and pain on micturition. There may be associated back pain.

Nursing management
This includes:
1. Obtaining a urine specimen for culture and sensitivity.
2. Administration of prescribed antibiotics and observation of patient for side effects, e.g. diarrhoea, allergic rash.
3. Encouraging patient to drink at least 3 litres daily.
4. Encouraging patient to empty bladder frequently (two- to four-hourly) and ensure complete emptying.
5. Educating patient about contributory factors.
6. Stressing importance of good hygiene practice, not wearing tight clothes around the perineum and avoiding the use of feminine deodorant sprays on the perineum.
7. Support and explanation to patient about further investigations to determine the cause of the infection, e.g. intravenous urogram, cystoscopy, bladder X-rays.

Pyelonephritis (acute)

Contributing factors as for cystitis. The bacteria reach the renal pelvis most commonly by reflux of urine from the bladder into the ureters (especially in children) and the commonest causative organism is *Escherichia coli*. The infection can arrive at the renal pelvis via the bloodstream and the causative organism then is often *Staphylococcus*.

The patient usually complains of fever, shivering, rigors, loin pain and tenderness, together with symptoms of cystitis, e.g. frequency, dysuria and strangury.

Nursing management
This includes the principles as for cystitis but as the patient will be generally unwell the following need to be taken into account:
1. Initially, the patient will need complete bed rest.
2. Prescribed analgesia will be required for relief of pain.
3. The patient will have a pyrexia and will require appropriate nursing measures to help reduce this.
4. Accurate observation and recording of urine output as well as fluid intake and assessment of patient for evidence of dehydration.

5. Observation of patient for complications of bed rest.

6. You would need to relate your care to the age and social circumstances of the patient. If this question is asked in relation to a 7-year-old girl, for example, then you would need to include appropriate care for a 7-year-old in hospital (see Chapter 3).

Chronic pyelonephritis is a common cause of chronic renal failure (discussed in 14.5, nephrotic syndrome). It is not usually a result of repeated acute attacks in an adult unless there has been a history of repeated acute attacks in childhood.

14.4. Specific care relating to patients having major surgery

General preoperative and postoperative care are discussed in Chapter 7, pp. 105–10. The notes below relate to specific points to be remembered when caring for patients undergoing the surgery indicated.

Renal

Specific preoperative investigations
1. Abdominal X-rays
2. Ultrasound
3. Intravenous urogram
4. Midstream specimen of urine or catheter specimen of urine
5. Twenty-four-hour urine collection, e.g. creatinine clearance, Ca^{2+}, PO_4^{3-} levels
6. Urinalysis, e.g. for blood, protein
7. Retrograde pyelogram
8. Renal biopsy
9. Renal arteriogram.

You should only include those relevant to the particular question you are answering in an examination as *all* investigations are not necessary prior to *all* renal surgery. For example, a renal biopsy and renal arteriogram are not necessary if a renal calculus has already been identified.

You should also indicate an understanding of why investigations are necessary and be able to identify the nurse's role in pre- and post-investigation care. For example, *specific nursing points* associated with
1. Renal biopsy:
(a) Explanation prior to procedure
(b) Availability of blood test results, e.g. anticoagulation studies
(c) Administration of sedation

(d) Position patient prone with pillow under abdomen

(e) Assist doctor with administration of local anaesthetic

(f) Explanation and reassurance to patient when needle is inserted, during X-ray to check position, and following removal of specimen applying pressure to site

(g) At least four hours complete bed rest and twenty-four hours lying flat in bed

(h) Quarter-hourly observations of pulse and blood pressure to detect early signs of haemorrhage for at least one hour then reduce frequency as condition permits

(i) Observation of urine for haematuria.

2. Intravenous urogram:

(a) Explanation prior to procedure

(b) Light diet day before

(c) Laxative on the evening before to clear intestines of gas and faeces

(d) Six to eight hours before the investigation, fluid restriction. If patient has had high fluid input then contrast medium is diluted and X-ray pictures may be unclear.

(e) No specific post-procedure care required, other than encouraging fluids especially if these were withheld prior to the procedure.

Specific aspects of postoperative management

These include:

1. Observations relating to airway and cardiovascular status should be made.

2. Observe dressing and pillows for evidence of haemorrhage.

3. Adequate, regular, intramuscular analgesia to relieve pain and allow patient to carry out deep breathing and coughing exercises which were taught preoperatively. These are vitally important to prevent respiratory complications but are painful because the surgical incision is close to the diaphragm, thus causing the patient to splint the chest when breathing.

4. Sit up and turn patient two-hourly to incision side to facilitate drainage and ease breathing.

5. Intravenous fluids initially. Encourage high oral intake when bowel sounds present.

6. If, following lithotomy, a nephrostomy tube is present, ensure it is draining properly. If ureteric catheter is present record drainage as instructed.

7. Accurate fluid balance chart must be maintained.

8. Advise on diet and good fluid intake in the future.

Prostatic: transurethral prostatectomy

Questions relating to prostatic surgery most commonly refer to the transurethral approach and involve elderly patients with chronic cardiac and/or respiratory problems. The care below relates specifically to patients undergoing a transurethral prostatectomy. Major points relating to the other approaches are discussed afterwards.

Specific preoperative care

This should relate to the information in the question about the patient, e.g. if they are *frail, elderly and suffer from chronic bronchitis* then care should include adequate nutritional build-up, including blood transfusion if anaemic, stopping smoking, encouraging deep breathing exercises, accurate fluid balance assessment.

In addition, the following should be considered: preparation, explanation and support for preoperative investigations, e.g. rectal examination, electrocardiograph, chest X-ray, possibly intravenous urogram, blood tests for urea, electrolyte, haemoglobin, grouping and cross-matching.

Specific postoperative care

1. Maintenance of airway
2. Observations to detect haemorrhage/shock
3. Relief of pain
4. Maintenance of accurate fluid balance chart for input, urine output and irrigation
5. Care of bladder irrigation:
(a) Three-way catheter
(b) Continuous drainage
(c) Observation of colour of flow, presence of clots
(d) Turning off irrigation and 'milking' catheter if obstructed
(e) Catheter care.
6. Encourage oral fluid intake when patient is able to tolerate oral fluids e.g. 3 litres in twenty-four hours.
7. Explain to patient purpose of irrigation, catheter, postoperative care.
8. Encourage early mobilization (NOT sitting for long periods).
9. Apply antiembolic stockings.
10. Administer postoperative antispasmodics if prescribed.
11. Try to keep stools soft by appropriate diet to prevent straining.
12. Explain to patient about regaining bladder control and teach appropriate perineal exercises.
13. Observe for evidence of urethral stricture, e.g. dysuria, small stream.

Notes relating to other approaches

These are most commonly suprapubic or retropubic, both of which require an abdominal incision (suprapubic also requires a bladder incision).

When the urethral catheter is removed leakage around the wound may occur, as may leakage around the suprapubic catheter site when this is removed following the suprapubic approach.

Bladder irrigation is not normally used following the retropubic approach. Otherwise specific care is as for transurethral approach.

14.5. Care relating to other renal problems

Acute renal failure

Key facts

1. Sudden onset causing oliguria or anuria
2. Caused by:
(a) Reduction in renal blood flow due, for example, to shock, haemorrhage, septicaemia, severe burns, arterial occlusion.
(b) Glomerular or tubular damage due, for example, to drugs, chemicals, haemoglobinuria
3. Two distinct clinical phases are present:
(a) Oliguric phase: urine output $\downarrow$ < 700 mls in twenty-four hours or $\downarrow$30 mls per hour; plasma urea $\uparrow$; K^+ $\uparrow$; $[H^+]$ $\uparrow$ $\therefore$ acidosis. Patient becomes drowsy, stuporous, nauseated and vomits.
(b) Diuretic phase: urine output $\uparrow$ up to 10 litres in twenty-four hours, therefore risk of dehydration with loss of H_2O and $\downarrow$ Na^+ and K^+. Gradually output returns to normal. Following this there is a return of urine output to normal, and the concentrating ability of the kidney also returns.

Treatment is directed at the primary cause and maintaining the patient's normal functions until spontaneous recovery occurs.

Key aspects of nursing management

1. Maintaining very accurate fluid balance chart
2. Daily weighing
3. Administering only the prescribed fluid intake, e.g. 500 mls + previous day's urine output volume
4. Giving patient low protein; low Na^+; low K^+; high carbohydrate diet
5. If K^+ levels high administering prescribed medication, e.g. calcium resonium rectally

6. If patient is nauseous and vomiting, administering prescribed fluids intravenously

7. Correctly administering peritoneal or haemodialysis if prescribed

8. When diuretic phase occurs observing for effects of dehydration and administering adequate fluids and electrolytes.

9. When caring for patients with acute renal failure it is vital that high potassium levels are detected early as cardiac arrhythmias may be caused leading to a cardiac arrest.

Because of the complicated biochemical monitoring of these patients, they are often transferred for dialysis to specialist units and you would not be expected to describe the care given in these situations in your final R.G.N. examination. If you are training in a hospital in which you gain experience in a renal unit, then it would be reasonable for the examiners in the internally set examination to expect you to discuss the care this type of patient requires.

Chronic renal failure (*uraemia*)

Key facts

1. Progressive, fatal condition unless patient is maintained on haemo-dialysis, or given a kidney transplant at an early stage of the renal disease process.

2. Decreased glomerular filtration occurs due to a decrease in number of functioning nephrons.

3. There are many causes including uncontrolled hypertension, chronic glomerulonephritis, chronic pyelonephritis, renal disease secondary to drug effects.

4. The onset is usually slow and associated with general malaise, nausea, vomiting, ↑ blood pressure, ↑ urea retention, polyuria, nocturia initially.

5. If treated very early with a low-protein diet deterioration can be stopped and the patient maintained for many years on strict diet.

6. If problems persist they become worse until all systems in the body are affected, e.g. drowsiness leading to coma; fits, oedema, weight loss, hypertension, pruritis, 'uraemic frost' on skin, osteoporosis, osteomalacia, acidosis.

Key aspects of nursing management

Nursing management of patients with chronic renal failure is related to treating their problems as they present. Careful maintenance of the diet –
↓ protein; ↓ Na^+ depending on serum levels; vitamin supplements,

adequate carbohydrate, fluid intake 500 mls plus previous day's urine volume is essential. They will be anaemic due to decreased ability to absorb iron and lack of production of erythropoietin. Administration of prescribed antihypertensive medication is important.

Ultimately, as the uraemic symptoms increase the nursing management becomes that of a terminally ill and unconscious patient, so nursing care needs to be directed towards ensuring the patient dies peacefully (see Chapter 19).

Nephrotic syndrome

Key facts
1. Causes include renal vein thrombosis and chronic glomerular nephritis.
2. It is a condition in which the glomerulus develops an increased permeability to proteins which causes proteinuria, reduced albumen levels and oedema.
3. There is always an increased serum cholesterol level.
4. The disease may progress to chronic renal failure.

Key aspects of nursing management
1. Bed rest initially
2. High-protein diet; ($\downarrow$ Na$^+$ if severe oedema)
3. Administration of prescribed medications which could include antibiotics, steroids, immunosuppressives and diuretics depending on the patient's condition
4. Care to prevent infection as patients are susceptible due to reduced plasma proteins, especially globulin
5. Specific care to prevent skin breakdown.

Acute glomerulonephritis

Key facts
1. This is an inflammatory reaction in the glomeruli.
2. Stimulus is often Group A streptococcal infection of the throat.
3. 'Complement' (aggregates of protein molecules) is formed as a result of the antigen–antibody reaction, become lodged in the glomeruli.
4. It occurs most commonly in children and young adults.
5. Initially, the disease present as oliguria or anuria, haematuria and proteinuria.
6. Other problems may include loin pain, fever, facial oedema and

headache, although some patients may have so mild an attack that they do not experience any of the above.

7. Complete recovery is normal, especially in children.

Key aspects of nursing management

1. Measurement and recording of accurate fluid input and urine output
2. Daily urinalysis for protein levels
3. Daily recording of patient's weight
4. Regular (four-hourly) observations of temperature, pulse, respiration and blood pressure to monitor trends of fever or hypertension.
5. Initial bed rest until proteinuria and haematuria decrease.
6. Throat swab to be taken for microscopy, culture and sensitivity and prescribed antibiotics administered.
7. Initially, fluids restricted, for example, 500 mls plus volume of previous day's urine output.
8. Diet − ↓ protein; ↓ Na^+ if oedema present; adequate carbohydrate. When diuresis occurs, e.g. after seven to ten days, fluids and protein can be increased. N.B. In the examination, if this question concerns a child remember to relate your care to the appropriate age group (see Chapter 3 for details).

Chronic glomerulonephritis

This is a form of the illness where repeated episodes of inflammation occur, causing severe damage to the kidneys. The associated high blood pressure causes circulatory problems and the patient may eventually develop chronic renal failure. The nursing management is directed at the problems the patient presents with and, in the later stages of the disease, these will include severe oedema, weight loss and cardiovascular problems.

14.6. Specimen R.G.N. questions

Q. 1. Mrs Ann Taylor, a young mother, is admitted to the ward with pyrexia and a history of recurrent cystitis. A diagnosis of acute pyelonephritis has been made.
(a) What factors may have led to the development of Mrs Taylor's condition?
(b) Describe the nursing care and treatment Mrs Taylor will require during her hospital stay.
    Final R.G.N. paper, English and Welsh National Board, March 1984

Q. 2. Mr John Evans, a 73-year-old retired railwayman, is fairly active despite a chronic chest condition and is to undergo a transurethral prostatectomy.

Explain how complications following Mr Evans's surgery can be prevented or detected by means of pre- and postoperative nursing care. 100%

Final R.G.N. paper, English and Welsh National Board, September 1984

14.7. Sample question and answer

Q. Mr Ian Townsend, a 70-year-old retired bus driver, who lives with his wife in local Part III accommodation, has been admitted for a transurethral prostatectomy. Using a problem-solving approach, describe in detail the postoperative care Mr Townsend will require during the first seventy-two hours. 100%

Problem	Nursing care/action
Difficulty with breathing	1. Ensure semi-prone position until conscious. 2. Observe respirations: depth, rate, rhythm, so as to detect respiratory problems. 3. Help to sit up in bed when conscious. 4. Encourage deep-breathing exercises. 5. Help with early mobilization (day 1 postoperatively)
Bladder irrigation via three-way Foley catheter	1. Ensure correctly connected and running easily. 2. Administer only prescribed fluids. 3. Observe flow for colour which will indicate amount of bleeding; rate which could indicate obstruction; presence of clots which could indicate an increase in rate or risk of obstruction. 4. Regulate flow rate as instructed to ensure clot retention is prevented. 5. If catheter stops draining, check tubing for kinks, 'milk' catheter and administer bladder washout if instructed. 6. Slow rate down as haematuria decreases and discontinue when instructed, e.g. after twenty-four to forty-eight hours.

Problem	Nursing care/action
Risk of haemorrhage from prostatic capsule	1. Carry out frequent observations of pulse and blood pressure initially, reducing to four-hourly when condition stable. 2. Observe urine colour for evidence of excessive haematuria. 3. Administer laxatives to avoid patient straining at stool.
Risk of urinary tract infection	1. Carry out catheter toilet four-hourly or more frequently if required. 2. Ensure good fluid intake, e.g. 2 to 3 litres daily. 3. Observe urine for evidence of infection – proteinuria, cloudy appearance, odour. 4. Send urine specimen for microscopy, culture and sensitivity after irrigation is discontinued. 5. Ensure trauma to urethra is minimized by correctly positioning catheter and drainage apparatus.
Pain	1. Administer prescribed analgesia regularly, as required, and assess effect, e.g. intramuscular Omnopon 15 mg four- to six-hourly during first forty-eight hours then oral aspirin and paraveretum six-hourly. 2. Help patient to achieve comfortable position in bed.
Immobility	1. Reposition patient two-hourly or help to change position when in bed. 2. Encourage early ambulation to prevent complications of bed rest. 3. Do not encourage patient to sit upright for prolonged periods as this increases intra-abdominal pressure and thus increases risk of haemorrhage. 4. Help patient to walk safely while irrigation is still in progress.
Difficulty maintaining hygiene	1. Wash face and hands when conscious and help patient change into clean pyjamas. 2. Offer mouthwashes as required. 3. Wash groin area as necessary. 4. Give bed bath first day postoperatively as patient will still have an intravenous infusion

Problem	Nursing care/action
	in one arm, may still feel drowsy due to the anaesthesia and will have bladder irrigation in progress.
	5. Help with washing as required on day 2 and day 3 until independent.
Difficulty with eating and drinking due initially to effects of anaesthetic	1. Nil orally until conscious and effects of anaesthetic have worn off.
	2. Give ice to suck or sips of water first, progressing to fluids if tolerated without nausea or vomiting.
	3. Give diet which will promote soft stools from day 1 postoperatively onwards.
Anxiety relating to	
(a) Hospitalization	1. Explain all nursing actions and care clearly to Mr Townsend.
	2. Take time to listen and talk to him about his worries.
(b) His wife	1. Ensure that his wife is able to visit and be flexible about visiting hours.
	2. Make the phone available for Mr Townsend to contact his wife.
	3. Reassure him that his wife is being looked after in their Part III accommodation by the warden.

The above answer could be presented in an essay form, but including clear identification of the problems associated with Mr Townsend's care. It would also be appropriate to include a short introductory paragraph if a care-plan format is to be used for the answer.

14.8. Multiple choice questions

Q. 1. If a patient is suffering from acute glomerulonephritis which one of the following groups of pathological results would be most likely:
(a) raised blood urea, raised serum sodium, reduced serum bicarbonate
(b) low blood urea, raised blood pressure, erythrocyte casts in the urine
(c) raised blood urea, raised blood pressure, lowered serum sodium
(d) raised blood urea, raised blood pressure, erythrocyte casts in the urine.

Because of glomerular damage, you would expect to find raised blood urea, raised blood pressure, raised sodium level and the presence of erythrocyte casts. Option (*b*) is incorrect because of reduced urea; option (*c*) is incorrect because of reduced sodium; and option (*a*) is incorrect because acidosis is not normally associated with acute glomerulonephritis. Thus (*d*) is the correct answer.

Q. 2. Which one of the following diets would be most suitable for a patient suffering from nephrotic syndrome?
(*a*) *high protein, restricted sodium with restricted fluid intake*
(*b*) *low protein, high carbohydrate with increased fluid intake*
(*c*) *high protein, low carbohydrate with restricted fluid intake*
(*d*) *low protein, restricted potassium with increased fluid intake.*

The most important aspects of a diet for a patient suffering from nephrotic syndrome are increased protein to replace the plasma proteins continually being lost, restricted fluids and a reduced sodium intake to help lessen the oedema. Options (*b*) and (*d*) are thus incorrect. Option (*c*) is also incorrect as an adequate, not reduced, carbohydrate intake is required. Option (*a*) is the correct answer.

15. Care of patients with gynaecological problems

15.1. Introduction

When caring for a patient with a gynaecological problem it is important to recognize and appreciate that the patient may have several different roles. She may be a wife, a mother with a family role to play, as well as being a partner and an individual.

A disorder of the female reproductive system will present many concerns for the individual in relation to the most personal and intimate aspects of their female sexuality. Many women have difficulty in talking about their problems because of embarrassment, fear or because to discuss such matters has been, and to some extent still is, socially unacceptable. Many gynaecological problems may cause a woman to feel inadequate and uncertain about her future relationships.

Investigations and treatment require the individual to reveal intimate facts and a part of her body which is usually private. The nurse should demonstrate sensitivity towards the patient's possible embarrassment and discomfort by ensuring privacy, support and confidentiality.

In caring for the person who has a gynaecological problem listening skills and empathy, as well as the ability to provide correct information and advice, are essential for the development of a trusting relationship between that person and the nurse.

Short notes are included in this chapter in relation to normal changes associated with pregnancy (15.2) and ante- and postnatal care (15.6).

15.2. Relevant anatomy and physiology

It is vital that a nurse has a good understanding of the anatomy and physiology of the female reproductive system so she can identify the physical problems a person with a disorder of the reproductive system may have. A knowledge of the physiological effects of the hormones also helps the nurse to understand some of the emotional changes that may occur in an individual as well as enabling her to give correct and appropriate advice to the patient about such hormonal effects.

It is outside the scope of this text to cover the above in sufficient detail for the examination requirements and students should refer to their lecture notes and an appropriate textbook for further details.

The following are the particular areas which students should include in their revision.

1. The structure of the uterus including the different types of tissue
2. The position of the uterus in the pelvis and how that position is maintained, including its relation to other organs, e.g. bladder, rectum, ureters
3. The menstrual cycle. Key aspects to include in this revision are:
(a) The three phases of the cycle – proliferative, secretory and menstrual
(b) How these phases relate to
(i) changes in the endometrium
(ii) secretion of hormones from the pituitary gland
(iii) ovarian production of oestrogen and progesterone
(iv) the ovarian cycle.
4. The normal changes associated with pregnancy which include:
amenorrhoea
'tingling heaviness' of breasts associated with enlargement
nausea and sickness (not necessarily in the morning)
urinary frequency and nocturia
constipation
emotional lability.

15.3. Key points relating to surgery

Hysterectomy

There are two main surgical approaches: abdominal or vaginal. Abdominal hysterectomy is usually carried out when the uterus is enlarged, e.g.

fibroids, or immobile due to adhesion and always when carcinoma of the body of the uterus is suspected. Vaginal hysterectomy is usually carried out when there are uterine problems, e.g. dysfunctional uterine bleeding, uterine prolapse and when the uterus is normal in size.

Specific aspects of nursing management
See Chapter 7 for general points.

Preoperative
1. Make appropriate skin preparations, e.g. lower abdominal and pubic shave.
2. Ensure bowels and bladder are emptied.
3. Give explanations of the operation and postoperative care, e.g. no abdominal wound if the vaginal approach is taken.
4. Listen and talk to the patient about her anxieties relating to her sexuality, self image or other specific fears, e.g. malignancy.
5. Educate the patient about the importance of postoperative exercises.
6. Collect midstream urine specimen and high vaginal swabs for detection of infection.
7. Ensure that blood has been taken for haemoglobin, full blood count, grouping and cross-matching of two units.

Postoperative
1. Management of urinary elimination: problems in voiding are not uncommon initially and catheterization is often used for the first three to four days and always following a vaginal hysterectomy.
2. Give care relating to vaginal pack if the vaginal approach was taken.
3. Observe blood loss on pads and record result.
4. Make an accurate record of fluid intake and output (intravenous infusion initially).
5. Encourage regular changes of position in bed and early ambulation.
6. Prevent complications associated with immobility: chest infections, deep vein thrombosis, constipation, urinary retention/stasis.
7. Advise as to when sexual intercourse can be resumed – usually after outpatient check-up and when the vault of the vagina has healed.
8. Advise the patient to contact her general practitioner if per vagina blood loss occurs. N.B. Remember to tell patient that she will no longer experience menstruation.
9. Discuss with her and her family the importance of rest, convalescence and no lifting, as well as how the family can best help her to recover her health.

10. Give advice on hormone replacement therapy if surgery has involved the removal of the ovaries and the patient is pre-menopause.

Colporrhaphy

Utero-vaginal prolapse occurs when one or more organs is displaced causing a bulge into the vagina. Most commonly this involves the bladder (*cystocele*) and rectum (*rectocele*).

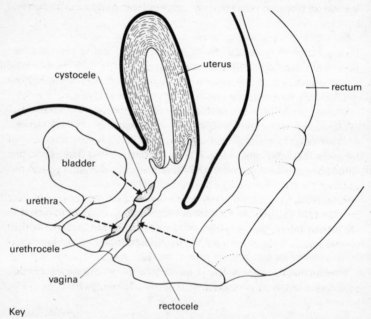

Key

— — — — → indicates direction of displacement

Both the above are normally associated with injuries received during childbirth although they may not appear until some years later. They can be caused by chronic coughing or as a result of increased abdominal pressure due, for example, to a cyst.

The problems they cause include incontinence, urgency, frequency in the case of a cystocele, and constipation in the case of a rectocele. The patient normally also complains of a 'nagging' backache.

There are two major procedures for the repair of the prolapse: anterior

colporrhaphy is the repair of the anterior vaginal wall, posterior colporrhaphy is the repair of the posterior vaginal wall.

Specific aspects of nursing management
Refer to Chapter 7 for general points.

Preoperative

Care is as for hysterectomy except that the explanations and support
should be directed towards the relief the woman will experience from her
specific problems and teaching of postoperative exercises, e.g. for perineal
muscles.

Postoperative

Care is as for a vaginal hysterectomy *but* special attention must be paid
to the prevention of infection. Vulval swabbing should be carried out
regularly, e.g. three times daily, until the patient is able to use the bidet.

The vaginal pack is removed twenty-four hours postoperatively and
analgesia, e.g. papaveretum 10 mg intramuscularly, should be given half
an hour prior to removal. Following removal, half-hourly recording of
the pulse rate and other observations to detect blood loss per vagina
should be made for four hours and the patient should remain on bed rest
to lessen the risk of secondary haemorrhage.

A normal diet can be given following a posterior repair but care
must be taken to prevent the patient becoming constipated. Exercises to
strengthen the perineal muscles should be encouraged, and the patient
should abstain from sexual intercourse, at least until her outpatient check-
up.

Explain that the repair will have *no* effect on menstruation or the ability
to conceive unless a hysterectomy has been performed as well.

15.4. Gynaecological emergencies (accidents of pregnancy)

Abortion

Therapeutic (legal) abortion can be carried out on the recommendation
of two medical practitioners in accordance with the 1967 Abortion Act –
students should refer to this for further details. If the patient is under 16
years, parental consent is required. Methods include suction termination
(normally at less than fourteen weeks) and prostaglandin termination.
Therapeutic abortion is usually a planned procedure not an emergency.

Spontaneous abortion can be divided into three categories: *threatened* is when the external cervical os remains closed and abortion can sometimes be prevented by bed rest and conservative treatment. It is associated with a slight brown loss per vagina and is usually painless. If this treatment fails then *inevitable* abortion will occur. *Incomplete* abortion is when some, but not all, of the foetus and placenta are expelled while some products of conception are retained in the uterus causing heavy blood loss per vagina and pain.

Key aspects of nursing management

1. Initially, maintain strict bed rest.
2. Give a normal diet with adequate fluids to avoid constipation and therefore straining which may induce contractions.
3. Administer prescribed medication, e.g. mild sedatives or myometrial relaxants, e.g. ritodrine.
4. When abortion becomes inevitable with increased vaginal blood loss, accurately observe and record the amount. Observe for signs of shock.
5. Withdraw food and oral fluids.
6. Administer and maintain intravenous fluids/blood transfusion.
7. Administer pain relief and assess effect.
8. Provide emotional support and *do not* leave patient alone.
9. Evacuation of the uterus is usually carried out under a general anaesthetic to ensure there are no retained products of conception.
10. Administer antibiotics as there is an increased infection risk.

All patients suffering a spontaneous abortion will experience an emotional reaction, the severity of which will depend upon their personality and particular circumstances. It is vitally important that the nurse is able to empathize with and care for patients in such a way as to help them overcome this experience.

They will require supportive counselling following the abortion and the nurse should refer them to appropriate agencies for help in the community following discharge, if they wish. The nurse should also explain to them the importance of not swimming, bathing, using tampons or having intercourse during the bleeding period following the abortion and reassure them that the bleeding should cease within one week.

They should be advised to seek medical advice if they develop a pyrexia, have very heavy bleeding or experience severe cramps.

Advice on future pregnancy should be given as appropriate, e.g. wait a couple of months for a full return to health.

Ectopic pregnancy

Key facts
1. This is a pregnancy in which the fertilized ovum fails to reach the uterus.
2. It normally becomes embedded in the Fallopian tube, which ruptures expelling the contents into the abdominal cavity between six and eight weeks after conception.

   The patient experiences severe abdominal pain when the rupture occurs followed by generalized abdominal pain.

   She also experiences signs of hypovolaemic shock due to haemorrhage, e.g. ↑ pulse, ↓ blood pressure, sweating, pallor.
3. Referred pain to the shoulder is experienced due to peritoneal irritation.
4. The only treatment is surgical intervention, which must be done quickly, as the condition is life-threatening.

Specific aspects of nursing management
1. Explain the need for surgery. Relatives can give consent if the patient is too ill.
2. Prepare for emergency laparotomy.
3. Administer and maintain fluids/blood transfusion to correct hypovolaemic shock.
4. Make frequent observations and record of patient's vital signs and general condition until taken to theatre which is often directly from the accident and emergency department.
5. Other preoperative care as indicated in Chapter 7.

   Postoperative care relates to that given to any patient following major abdominal surgery but specific counselling will be required in relation to the emotional effects of the emergency. The patient may have been trying desperately to become pregnant and thus will experience the same 'loss' reaction as if she had had a spontaneous abortion.

15.5. Infertility

If you are asked about this topic it is most likely to be as part of a question or as a question requiring an essay-style answer.

   The points listed below are those you should include in your revision.
1. Initial assessment.
(a) Involve both partners.
(b) Are they having full intercourse?

(c) How often are they having intercourse?

(d) How long has she been trying to get pregnant?

(e) What are their feelings about having children?

2. Specific information required from the female partner includes:

(a) menstrual history: stated periods, regularity, length of cycle

(b) age

(c) any previous relevant illnesses/operations, e.g. pelvic inflammatory disease, ovarian cysts, appendicitis, tuberculosis

(d) any medication which may affect fertility.

3. Specific information from male partner includes:

(a) any medication which may affect fertility

(b) any relevant operations

(c) does he ejaculate during intercourse?

(d) did he have mumps in childhood?

4. Further investigations.

(a) Temperature chart to pinpoint ovulation (temperature ↑) and thus the couple to increase frequency of intercourse at this time

(b) Sperm count after intercourse – i.e. intercourse should take place the night before they go to the clinic

(c) Laparoscopy for female partner to visualize ovaries and Fallopian tubes

(d) Dilatation and curettage to assess phase of endometrium

(e) Blood specimens for F.S.H. and L.H. blood levels

(f) Dye techniques, e.g. hysterosalpingogram to show up Fallopian tubes

(g) Drug therapy to induce ovulation.

Once a couple is definitely known to be infertile the following options exist:

1. Accept the fact and make a life together without their own children – ? increased involvement with the children of friends or relatives.

2. Seek adoption or fostering.

3. Try artificial insemination if male partner is sterile.

4. Seek support from marriage guidance counsellor and Childless Couples Association.

15.6. Health education issues and pregnancy

This section includes key points you would be expected to include in discussion answers on the topics covered below. Health education is directed at healthy as well as ill people in order to encourage them to take an interest in their own wellbeing and health promotion. Students should be becoming increasingly familiar with this aspect of nursing care and it is likely to form a much greater part of examination questions in the future.

Ante- and postnatal care are included here because pregnancy is a normal healthy condition. The objectives of antenatal care are to promote the health and wellbeing of the mother and unborn child and to prevent complications of pregnancy by early detection of problems and good health education for the mother. The objectives of postnatal care are to prevent possible complications following birth and to promote the wellbeing of the mother and child.

The current R.G.N. syllabus does not expect students to have a detailed knowledge of obstetric care but it does expect them to have a basic understanding of the principles involved in care and the importance of these.

Antenatal care

Following confirmation of pregnancy by her general practitioner the woman will first attend the hospital at a 'booking' antenatal clinic. This visit is crucially important to the mother as it provides her first experience of what antenatal care is, and the impression that she gains from this visit will determine how she views the rest of her pregnancy. It is important that she feels *involved* in her care and the nurse needs to explain clearly any clinical procedures and the woman's right to refuse. The atmosphere must be caring and help the woman to feel at ease and be able to discuss her questions and anxieties. The antenatal clinic should be a forum where she can meet other mothers and children, discuss her problems and develop a trusting relationship with those who will be supporting her during her pregnancy.

The following should be included in the initial assessment of the mother:
1. Present health status
(a) Is she taking any medication?
(b) Does she smoke/drink alcohol?
(c) Does she feel well?
(d) Has she had any health problems in the past, e.g. epilepsy, diabetes, high blood pressure, depression?
2. Assessment of vital signs
(a) blood pressure for evidence of hypertension
(b) temperature to indicate possible infection.
3. Urinalysis
(a) Sugar may indicate diabetic response to pregnancy.
(b) Protein may indicate infection.

(c) Ketones may indicate diabetes or poor eating habits.

4. Full medical examination which includes examination of the breasts, may include an internal examination, and blood tests for haemoglobin, blood group, rubella titre and Wasserman reaction.

5. Advice will need to be given to the mother in relation to:

(a) diet, e.g. the importance of vitamin D intake for Asian woman;

(b) weight: the need to monitor weight regularly during pregnancy;

(c) lifting: advise not to lift heavy weights and teach good lifting technique;

(d) shoes: feet enlarge during pregnancy, thus comfortable shoes with low heels should be worn to help with posture and prevent backache;

(e) benefits: e.g. maternity benefit and grant, milk allowances and free dental treatment;

(f) antenatal clinics: frequency, next appointment, reasons for attendance.

Topics which can be discussed at antenatal classes include breast-feeding, pain relief, the delivery, relaxation techniques. These discussions should also involve the father whenever possible and serve as an opportunity for the couple to meet other prospective parents. The mother should feel able to discuss matters which arise in antenatal classes when she attends her antenatal appointments at the clinic.

During the pregnancy the nurse must explain the necessity for various procedures, e.g. ultrasound scanning and the importance of regular monitoring of weight and blood pressure and the further collection of blood and urine specimens.

It is important that the mother can look forward to antenatal care and become interested in it as she and her husband are much more likely to gain full benefit from the advice and support that is offered.

Postnatal care

Key points to consider are:

1. assessment of bleeding per vagina
2. observation of stitches following episiotomy or perineal tear
3. monitoring of temperature for indication of infection
4. encouraging fluids and diet
5. checking to ensure no problems with passing urine or having bowels open
6. pain relief especially if severe 'after pains'
7. adequate rest
8. advice and explanations on breast-feeding and bottle-feeding; care of baby; tests, e.g. Guthrie; bonding; contraception; ?need for support at

home; role of domiciliary midwife; role of health visitor; needs of the rest of the family; follow-up appointments and care.

Cervical screening

This is a very important area for health educators as early detection and treatment of cervical changes can prevent development of carcinoma of the cervix.

The greatest problem encountered in health education is to convince women that it really is in their best interests to have regular cervical smears (frequency depending on the previous smear results).

Places where cervical smears can be carried out are included in the sample answer on pp. 258–9.

Persons/agencies involved in educating women about this are:

1. Health care professionals: general practitioners; health visitors; district nurses; midwives; hospital nurses; family planning clinic nurses; school nurses.
2. The government via campaigns organized nationally through the Department of Health and Social Security; this includes pamphlet and poster distribution as well as radio and television advertising
3. Voluntary agencies: women's organizations; charities; women's self-help groups
4. The media: radio programmes; television documentaries; newspaper articles and reports; women's magazines
5. Health centres through information documents, lectures and discussions and health education videos.

Other issues to consider are:

1. a national computer register of all women and their smear results;
2. local register organized by general practitioners;
3. mandatory cervical smears for all women over a certain age.

N.B. The ways in which the health professionals are involved is discussed in the sample answer on pp. 258–9.

15.7. Specimen R.G.N. question

Q. Miss Dorothy Thompson, a 55-year-old school-teacher who lives alone, has a two-year history of menorrhagia. She is apprehensive, having just been admitted to undergo vaginal hysterectomy.

(a) What nursing measures may be taken to alleviate Miss Thompson's anxiety and prepare her psychologically for operation?   30%

(*b*) *Outline the care Miss Thompson will require during the first seventy-two hours postoperatively and the information junior nursing staff will need to enable them to understand its relevance.*   70%

Final R.G.N. Paper, English and Welsh National Board, January 1985

15.8. Sample question and answer

Q. Mrs Elizabeth Evans, aged 38 years, married with two teenage children, is admitted to your ward for radium implant therapy for carcinoma of the cervix. The diagnosis was made after she had a cervical smear taken at her local 'well woman' clinic.
(*a*) *Discuss the availability of cervical screening and the role of nurses in making women more aware of the need for regular cervical smears.* 50%

(*b*) *Describe the specific nursing management Mrs Evans will require, following the insertion of a radioactive source until its removal forty-eight hours later.*   50%

(*a*) A discussion of availability should include identifying the places where cervical smears can be taken and whether these facilities are commonly known about or readily available to all women. The places identified should include: general practitioners' surgeries; family planning clinics; well-woman clinics; sexually-transmitted-disease clinics; private screening agencies; hospitals including antenatal, postnatal and gynaecological outpatient clinics.

A discussion of the way in which nurses are involved should include the roles of
1. the *school nurse* in educating teenage girls about the need for regular cervical smears after they have become sexually active and the special importance of this if they have been having intercourse for some years already;
2. the *family planning nurse* in asking her clients about when they last had a smear, discussing with them the need for regular smears, and, where appropriate, taking a smear;
3. the *district nurse* in identifying patients who may be in need of cervical smears and encouraging them to have these taken, e.g. an elderly lady with an offensive vaginal discharge or vaginal bleeding. The district nurse should educate all her female patients about the need for regular cervical smears and she can either suggest they visit their general practitioner or give them details of where they could go for a smear to be taken.

4. the *hospital nurse* in counselling and advising all the women that she looks after and works with about the need for cervical smears; she is often in a position to arrange for it to be done in the hospital if the woman so wishes while she is still an inpatient.

5. Obstetric nurses and midwives in ensuring that clients are given appropriate advice in relation to cervical smears and understand the need for these to be carried out.

All nurses have a responsibility to educate members of the public about health issues and should do so when the appropriate opportunity arises. They should also ensure that they set a role model example by attending for regular cervical screening themselves.

(*b*) The question asks only for *specific* care and does not require you to discuss either the care required during insertion or removal.

The following aspects of nursing management should be included:

1. Safety of staff and visitors:

(a) Ensure staff wear radiation detection badges.

(b) Don't allow children or pregnant women to enter the room.

(c) Only spend time in the room for essential nursing duties not just 'chatting' to Mrs Evans.

(d) Ensure lead box and long-handled forceps are available in the room for use if required, e.g. if the source becomes dislodged.

(e) The source should only be handled with forceps.

(f) Limit the amount of time visitors spend in the room.

(g) When carrying out care try to remain as far as practicably possible away from the source.

(h) Do not carry out perineal care.

2. Reducing Mrs Evans's anxiety in relation to the procedure and the 'isolation' in a cubicle.

(a) Explain clearly the reason for the isolation.

(b) Ensure she knows it is only for forty-eight hours.

(c) When carrying out nursing duties use the time to talk to Mrs Evans and listen to her fears and anxieties.

(d) Provide aids to help her occupy her time, e.g. books, radio, television.

3. Maintain Mrs Evans's comfort by supporting her with pillows in bed and turning her from side to side as required. She will be on strict bed rest.

4. Prevent complications due to bed rest.

5. Observe the applicator for evidence of dislodgement – it should be well secured with vaginal packing.

6. Observe and record urinary output via the catheter.

7. Monitor temperature and general condition for evidence of infection.

16. Care of patients with blood-related disorders and oncological nursing management

16.1. Introduction 16.2. Anatomy and physiology: constituents of blood; formation and destruction of red blood cells; clotting; blood groups 16.3. Blood transfusion 16.4. Severe haemorrhage 16.5. Blood disorders: anaemia; leukaemia 16.6. Management of patients undergoing oncological treatment: chemotherapy; radiotherapy; carcinoma of the breast 16.7. Specimen R.G.N. questions 16.8. Sample question and answer

16.1. Introduction

This chapter describes the constituents of blood and the formation and destruction of red blood cells. Specific care of patients receiving a blood transfusion and care relating to severe haemorrhage, e.g. ruptured spleen, is also included. The major blood disorders are summarized and the specific aspects of nursing management listed.

Notes relating to the care of patients requiring oncological nursing are included in this chapter as it was felt that to include all notes relating to this topic in one chapter was more helpful for revision purposes than to include only those aspects relevant to the care of patients with leukaemia. Specific care relating to management of patients with carcinoma of the breast is thus included in this chapter.

16.2. Anatomy and physiology

Constituents of blood

Key facts
1. It contains white blood cells, red blood cells, plasma and platelets.
2. Red blood cells (*erythrocytes*) contain haemoglobin, have no nucleus and have a lifespan of approximately 120 days. Their main function is to

transport oxygen from the lungs to the tissues, and there are approximately 5 million red cells per mm^3 of blood.

3. White blood cells (*leucocytes*) have a nucleus and are larger than red cells. Their lifespan is twenty to thirty days. Of the different types *granulocytes* are the most numerous and include mostly *neutrophils* with some *eosinophils* and *basophils*. The two types found mostly in the peripheral circulation are *lymphocytes* and *monocytes*.

4. Neutrophils are phagocytic and contain enzymes to digest bacteria. Eosinophils have an antihistamine effect. Basophils contain histamine and heparin. The main role of lymphocytes is in immunity and monocytes are phagocytic.

5. Platelets (*thrombocytes*) have no nucleus, are smaller than red blood cells and have a half life of approximately seven days. They are formed from *megakaryocytes* in the bone marrow and are destroyed in the spleen. They collect at the site of injury and form a sticky 'plug' as well as releasing serotonin which assists vasoconstriction.

6. The above are suspended in the plasma which is 90 per cent water and contains plasma proteins, NaCl, HCO$_3$ and other transported substances, e.g. vitamins, glucose, hormones.

7. If blood is left to stand and clotting prevented, it separates into three layers – plasma on top, white cells in the middle and red cells at the bottom.

8. The percentage of red cells by volume is known as the *haematocit* (packed cell volume). The normal is 45 per cent. An ↑ haematocit indicates ↓ plasma volume or ↑ circulating red cells and a ↓ haematocit indicates ↑ plasma volume or ↓ circulating red cells.

9. If whole blood is allowed to clot and the clot removed the remaining fluid is called *serum*.

Formation and destruction of red blood cells

Formation occurs in adults only in the red bone marrow pulp. It is under the control of the hormone erythropoietin. The erythropoietin promotes the differentiation of the appropriate committed stem cells to form proerythroblasts.

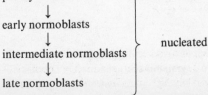

proerythroblasts
↓
early normoblasts
↓
intermediate normoblasts   nucleated
↓
late normoblasts

↓

reticulocytes (nucleus degenerating)

↓

erythrocytes (NO nucleus)

In addition to erythropoietin other factors controlling red cell production are vitamin B_{12} folic acid and iron.

Erythrocytes are destroyed in the reticuloendothelial system. The iron from the haem portion is stored for re-use while the rest of the haem is converted first to biliverdin and then bilirubin for excretion in the bile. The globin portion and cell portion are broken down to amino acids.

Clotting

You should not be expected to know all the factors involved in the process but you should be able to summarize the effects: for example,

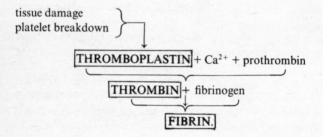

tissue damage
platelet breakdown

THROMBOPLASTIN + Ca^{2+} + prothrombin

THROMBIN + fibrinogen

FIBRIN.

Fibrinogen is a soluble plasma protein present in the blood.

Fibrin is insoluble.

Factor VIII (antihaemophilic globulin) catalyses the reaction in which the loose fibrin strands form a dense fibrin network in the presence of Ca^{2+}.

Clotting normally occurs within about ten minutes.

Heparin inhibits prothrombin → thrombin. Warfarin inhibits formation of prothrombin in the liver. Aspirin decreases platelet stickiness.

Blood groups

The antigens on the surface of red cells are called *agglutinogens*. Antibodies against agglutinogens are called *agglutinins* and are found in the plasma. Agglutination occurs between *donor* cells and *recipient* plasma.

Blood group	O	A	B	AB
Cells	no agglutinogen	A agglutinogen	B agglutinogen	A and B agglutinogens
Plasma	anti-A and anti-B agglutinins	anti-B agglutinin	anti-A agglutinin	no agglutinins

Group AB is the universal recipient.
Group O is the universal donor.

DONOR	GROUP	RECIPIENTS

Eighty-five per cent of the population also have agglutinogen D and are referred to as Rhesus-positive. The other 15 per cent are Rhesus-negative. Anti-D can *only* be formed by Rhesus-negative people after sensitization with Rhesus-positive blood.

A person with Anti-D subsequently transfused with D-positive blood may develop a severe transfusion reaction. If a Rhesus-negative mother becomes sensitized and has a Rhesus-positive foetus then the anti-D can cross the placenta and may cause the death of the baby due to agglutination and haemolysis.

16.3. Blood transfusions

The important aspects of nursing management concern the measures taken to avoid the hazards associated with blood transfusion and the early detection of complications.

These are:

1. *Haemolytic reaction* due to incompatibility. It is to avoid this that prior to administration the details relating to grouping, cross-matching and expiry date are checked to ensure they are the same on the blood bag and in the documentation and that they relate to the patient to whom the transfusion has been given. Severe reactions usually start within the first twenty minutes following commencement of the transfusion. Initially, the patient may complain of low backache, chills and a headache but if the transfusion is not stopped then fever, hypotension and collapse will follow.

2. *Circulatory overload* can occur especially if the patient is elderly or suffers from heart failure and whole blood is being transfused. The patient should have frequent observations of respiratory rate and depth made and he should be observed for evidence of dyspnoea, cyanosis or a productive cough.

3. *Febrile reaction* can be due to the presence of bacteria, but this is normally avoided by correct storage (4° C) and use of bacterial filters. Sensitivity to leucocytes or platelets in the transfused blood may cause a gradual rise in temperature during transfusion but this normally resolves itself afterwards without other serious effects.

4. *Allergic reactions* usually cause the patient to complain of itching and to develop urticaria. This may be due to sensitivity to a plasma protein in the transfused blood.

Correct aseptic technique for inserting the cannula, changing units of blood and the administration set, as well as observing the cannula site regularly for evidence of misplacement or inflammation all contribute to avoid *thrombophlebitis, air-embolism* and *septicaemia.*

Whole blood is normally *only* given to patients who are acutely bleeding or suffering from hypovolaemic shock due to haemorrhage.

Packed cells are given in most other cases as they produce a lesser volume load on the circulation but still contain the same amount of red cells as a unit of whole blood.

16.4. Severe haemorrhage

Severe haemorrhage can occur as a result of trauma or in association with a disease process. Nursing management is directed towards stopping the bleeding where possible, maintaining the airway and blood replacement régime and preparing the patient for appropriate surgical intervention.

Specific aspects of nursing management

The points below relate to a patient with a ruptured spleen but the principles are applicable to any major haemorrhage with associated hypovolaemia.

1. Maintaining airway:
(a) Semi-prone position
(b) Frequent observation of respiratory depth, rate and rhythm
(c) Observing of respiratory complications, e.g. dyspnoea.
2. Monitoring haemodynamic state:
(a) Observing and recording quarter- to half-hourly: pulse rate, volume and rhythm; blood pressure.
(b) Recording central venous pressure if line *in situ*
(c) Observing skin colour, temperature.
3. Maintaining blood replacement:
(a) Initially group O Rh-negative blood or plasma substitute, e.g. Haemaccel
(b) Correctly grouped and cross-matched blood when available.
4. Other care, e.g. observation for other injuries; girth measurements; administering prescribed analgesia; obtaining information about patient from friends or relatives if possible; assisting medical staff with examination, taking blood specimens for grouping, cross-matching and full blood count.

Normal preoperative preparation and safety checks would be made but in answer to an examination question you must show the examiner that you appreciate that this is an emergency and concentrate on the important aspects only.

16.5. Blood disorders

Anaemia

Key facts

There are two main groups of anaemias:
1. Those associated with reduced red blood cell production by the bone marrow and these include:
(a) iron deficiency which is the commonest cause of anaemia
(b) vitamin B_{12} deficiency and folic acid deficiency due to a lack in dietary intake
(c) vitamin B_{12} (extrinsic factor) deficiency as a result of a lack of intrinsic factor in the gastric juice which is called pernicious anaemia

(d) aplastic, which is usually a result of bone marrow depression or destruction caused by a reaction to certain drugs, e.g. chloramphenicol; radiation damage; benzene-based chemicals and other toxic agents.

2. Those associated with excessive destruction of red blood cells (haemolytic) and these include:
(a) sickle cell
(b) other hereditary red blood cell deficiencies, e.g. spherocytosis
(c) thalassaemia major
(d) autoimmune.

A patient suffering from pernicious anaemia has a red tongue which is smooth and sore.

The extrinsic factor cannot be absorbed in the ileum without the intrinsic factor being present.

Patients suffering from aplastic and haemolytic anaemias will often require reverse barrier nursing during crises because of their susceptibility to infection. They will also require blood transfusion.

Nursing management

This is directed at the problems of which individual patients complain, including fatigue, general weakness, breathlessness on exertion, headache, insomnia, anorexia, dyspepsia, palpitations and increased heart rate. Patients require support and explanations concerning treatment and investigation, e.g. bone marrow aspiration.

Where appropriate, dietary advice and education should be given as well as explanation about the importance of taking prescribed medication regularly.

If answering a question relating to care of an elderly person then details as in Chapter 6 should be included as necessary.

Leukaemia

Key facts

Leukaemia is a malignant disorder in which there is an accumulation of white blood cells in bone marrow and peripheral blood.

It can be an acute or chronic illness.

1. *Acute* leukaemias have an onset over weeks or days rather than months and involve immature malignant cells. *Acute lymphoblastic* is most commonly seen in children and *acute myeloid* in adults.

In the bone marrow there is:
$\downarrow$ red cell production $\rightarrow$ anaemia
$\downarrow$ platelet production $\rightarrow$ bleeding

↓ normal white blood cells → infection

↑ abnormal white blood cells

Treatment consists of chemotherapy:

(a) Induction and maintenance

(b) Prompt treatment of infection

(c) Transfusion of blood, platelets and white blood cells

(d) Bone marrow transplantation in some cases.

2. *Chronic* leukaemias have an insidious onset over months or years and involve differentiated malignant cells.

Chronic myeloid is seen in young to middle-aged adults mostly and they may complain of left upper abdominal pain due to an enlarged spleen, general non-specific weakness and malaise. In the later stages, the spleen enlarges, anaemia increases, bone pain develops and haemorrhaging may occur. Chronic myeloid normally develops into acute myeloid which is resistant to treatment.

Chronic lymphocytic is the commonest form of leukaemia and is mostly seen in adults over 50 years of age. It is often discovered as a result of routine blood tests in an otherwise well person. It is associated with a slightly enlarged spleen, painful lymph nodes and a marked tendency to infection due to an inability to synthesize antibodies. Autoimmune haemolytic anaemia may develop.

Treatment for both chronic myeloid and chronic lymphocytic leukaemia consists of chemotherapy, possible irradiation of the spleen; for lymphocytic, irradiation of the lymph nodes to provide symptomatic relief.

Key aspects of nursing management

1. Appropriate preparation, explanation and care relating to (a) chemotherapy and (b) radiotherapy (see 16.6).

2. Specific care relating to:

(a) increased risk of infection

(b) increased bleeding tendency

(c) problems caused by the anaemia.

3. Psychological support for the patient and family.

4. Care related to the many associated problems, e.g. pain, pyrexia, sweating, anorexia, weight loss, fatigue and general malaise.

Further details are included in the sample answer.

16.6. Management of patients undergoing oncological treatment

Chemotherapy

You would not be expected to know details about specific chemotherapeutic agents but you should familiarize yourself with those commonly in use in your hospital and you should know the general side effects.

Specific aspect of nursing care

1. *Prior to treatment*: explanation and teaching of patient and family about the drugs and the side effects.
2. *After treatment*: care associated with the side effects and problems the patient may experience.

(a) Nausea and vomiting:
   (i) Give antiemetics $\pm$ sedatives.
   (ii) Give food at times when not nauseous, in small attractive portions.

(b) Stomatitis (occurs approximately two weeks after chemotherapy): four- to six-hourly mouth care to prevent deterioration in the mucous membrane lining.

(c) Diarrhoea:
   (i) Low residue diet
   (ii) Antidiarrhoeal drugs.

(d) Risk of infection (due to suppression of white blood cell production):
   (i) Good hand-washing technique for patient and all staff
   (ii) Reverse barrier nursing
   (iii) Four-hourly temperature recording.

(e) Risk of bleeding (due to thrombocytopaenia):
   (i) Avoid intramuscular injections
   (ii) Observe for bleeding
   (iii) Record blood pressure and pulse regularly
   (iv) Care when lifting or moving patient
   (v) Stop use of toothbrush
   (vi) Administer and maintain platelet infusions
   (vii) Pad bed rails; use bed cradles.

(f) Fatigue (due to $\uparrow$ urea and uric acid as a result of breakdown of cancer cells):
   (i) Promote comfort and rest
   (ii) Prevent over-exertion.

(g) Alopecia:
   Provide a wig if required.

Radiotherapy

Specific aspects of nursing care
1. Explanation of treatment and procedures and visit to department for patient prior to treatment.
2. Educate patient about precautions to take:
(a) Do not apply ointments, creams, cosmetics to site
(b) Wear loose-fitting clothes
(c) Keep skin area dry and exposed if possible
(d) Avoid extremes of temperature and sunshine
(e) *DO NOT* rub off radiologist's markings.
3. Ensure good nutritious diet with adequate fluid intake.
4. Promote comfort and rest.
5. Problems associated with radiotherapy include: bleeding gums, dry mouth, anorexia, nausea, vomiting, weakness, fatigue, tender skin, irritation, local hair loss.
6. Provide psychological support for treatment and self-image.
7. Include care specific to the particular site, e.g. the patient's difficulty with swallowing if neck, chest irradiated.

Carcinoma of the breast

This topic is included here as surgery to the breast is almost always carried out for carcinoma and it is a subject with which the examiners would expect you to be familiar.

Key facts
1. This is the most common malignancy in women.
2. It is a major cause of death in women.
3. The patient usually has no obvious physiological problems.
4. A 'lump' is discovered following self-examination or attendance at the general practitioner's surgery or clinic.
5. Specific tests may include mammography, thermography, biopsy, aspiration of breast tissue.

Specific preoperative preparation
1. Assist patient to come to terms with diagnosis.
2. Explain the surgical procedures.
3. Discuss with patient and family the postoperative appearance of her chest, their expectation of surgery, altered self-image and other anxieties the patient may have, e.g. fear of death.

4. Arrange appropriate counselling and referral as for any patient with malignant disease.
5. Shave axilla.
6. Normal preoperative preparation.

Specific postoperative care
 1. Adequate pain relief
 2. Comfortable positioning: sitting up with arm on the operated side well supported or in a sling
 3. Regular arm exercises after first forty-eight hours
 4. Observation and care of wounds, drains, skin flaps
 5. Reinforcement of preoperative teaching and counselling
 6. Helping patient to accept changed body image
 7. Involvement of family in discussions and care
 8. Arranging referrals for, e.g., sexual counselling; Mastectomy Association; fitting of prosthesis
 9. Teaching self-examination of breasts
10. Information about further treatment – radiotherapy or chemotherapy – and help patient to understand the effects of this.
11. Give advice about convalescence to include:
(a) Avoidance of heavy lifting
(b) Regular exercises
(c) Need to experience grieving
(d) Care relating to prosthesis
(e) Importance of outpatient department follow-up.

16.7. Specimen R.G.N. questions

Q.1. (a) *What are the hazards of blood transfusion and what measures should be taken to avoid them?*   40%

   Martin, an 18-year-old student, has been admitted in a state of shock after an accident on the rugby field. A diagnosis of ruptured spleen has been made.
(b) *Describe the nursing care Martin will need prior to surgery.*   60%

Final R.G.N. examination, English and Welsh National Board, November 1984

Q.2. (*a*) *Give a brief account of the ways in which the body limits haemor-rhage.*   20%

Ann Jones, a 17-year-old schoolgirl, has been admitted to hospital follow-ing repeated heavy nosebleeds. The current episode is being controlled with icepacks. She has been received into a four-bedded bay.
(*b*) *Outline a plan of care, for a period of 24 hours, with particular reference to Ann's:*
(*i*) *bleeding*   40%
(*ii*) *discomfort*   25%
(*iii*) *anxiety*   15%

Final R.G.N. examination, English and Welsh National Board, January
1984

16.8. Sample question and answer

Ian Peters, a 22-year-old university student, has recently been diagnosed as having acute myeloid leukaemia.
(*a*) *Using a problem-solving approach describe Ian's management and care during his first week in hospital.*   75%

(*b*) *How may Ian and his family be helped to accept his prognosis?* 25%

(a) Key points to include in the answer are:

Problem	Nursing action
Increased risk of infection	1. Reverse barrier nursing.
	2. Good hand-washing technique for use by staff and patient.
	3. Exclude infected persons from contact and limit visitors.
	4. Record temperature and pulse four-hourly.
	5. Observe for other signs of infection, e.g. phlebitis, abscesses.
	6. Collect appropriate specimens and send to laboratory for microscopy, culture and sensitivity at regular intervals.
	7. Encourage adequate fluids and nutritious diet.
	8. Give special attention to caring for intravenous site.

Problem	Nursing action
Increased bleeding tendency	1. Observe for bleeding, e.g. gums, nose, stools. 2. Avoid intramuscular injections. 3. Record blood pressure and pulse regularly. 4. Lift and move patients with caution. 5. Stop use of toothbrush. 6. Administer/maintain platelet infusions safely. 7. Pad bed rails; use bed cradles.
Nausea and vomiting	1. Give prescribed antiemetic and sedative drugs and assess effect. 2. Be flexible with mealtimes. 3. Encourage foods which do not have a nauseous effect. 4. Provide vomit bowl and tissues within easy reach.
Pain	1. Try to ensure comfortable position. 2. Administer prescribed analgesia in small amounts regularly to control pain.
Anaemia, causing weakness lethargy dyspnoea	1. Encourage patient to rest. 2. Administer/maintain blood transfusion safely. 3. Prevent over-exertion. 4. Ensure comfortable, well-supported position. 5. Give appropriate dietary supplements.
Anorexia	1. Offer small appetizing meals. 2. Find out Ian's preferences and try to make these available or encourage family to bring food in for him.
Anxiety in relation to: isolation due to reverse barrier nursing and visiting restrictions	1. Explain fully reasons for isolation and restrictions. 2. Try to ensure 'key nurse' relationship is allowed to develop with Ian and his family.
hospitalization chemotherapy	3. Orientate him to hospital and ward. 4. Explain about chemotherapy.
Anxiety about prognosis: see (b).	

(b) Points to include in this section are:
1. Development of trusting relationship
2. Honest communication

3. Discussion of fears with Ian and his family together
4. Referral to other counsellors where appropriate, e.g. priest, specialist cancer counsellor
5. Support for all the family in relation to coping with feelings of guilt and potential loss
6. Involvement of all family members in group support
7. Good clear explanations of treatment goals and involvement in planning Ian's care
8. Listening to Ian and his family as well as talking to them.

In answering part (a) it is important to remember you are only asked about the first week of care and thus undue emphasis should not be placed on the side effects of chemotherapy which would only become serious when bone marrow suppression occurred approximately two weeks after treatment. The answer could be written easily in an essay form with identification of the problems. The plan style used above is to highlight points to consider when revising the subject.

17. Immunization and care of patients with infection

17.1. Introduction

The nurse has an important role to play, both in the hospital and the community, in the promotion of childhood immunization programmes and health education in relation to good hygiene and the prevention of infection.

Preventing infection spreading is of considerable importance especially in hospital wards where patients are often already more susceptible to infection as a result of pre-existing illness.

You are advised to read current research and infection control literature, as the role of the nurse in this area is a topic which may be considered for inclusion in the longer type of question in the internally set examination during the transition period.

Key points relating to asepsis are included in Chapter 7.

17.2. Childhood immunization

Immunity can be acquired in four different ways:
1. *natural active* by production of antibodies in response to a disease or infection which the person has acquired;
2. *natural passive* by transfer of antibodies from the mother to her foetus via the placenta or to her baby via breast secretions;
3. *artificial active* by introduction of a bacterial or viral preparation into the body which stimulates the body to produce antibodies;
4. *artificial passive* by injection of serum containing antibodies that have been produced in another host.

Childhood vaccination programme

3 to 6 months: whooping cough, diphtheria, tetanus; polio vaccine.
   Whooping cough (pertussis), diphtheria and tetanus vaccine are given together and known as 'triple vaccine'.
5 months: triple vaccine and polio vaccine.
11 months: triple vaccine and polio vaccine.
   An interval of approximately two months should elapse between the initial and second vaccination and a further four to six months before the third vaccination. Thus, the ages given above will vary depending on individual circumstances.
12 to 24 months: measles vaccine.
5 years: diphtheria, tetanus; polio vaccine booster. This can be given on entry to nursery school but is normally given at least three years after completion of the basic course.
10 to 13 years: B.C.G. vaccine; rubella vaccine (for girls only).
15 years: polio, tetanus vaccine booster. This is normally given ten years after the previous booster.
   It is not compulsory for any of the above vaccinations to be given. It is therefore crucially important that nurses take an active role in educating the public about the importance of prevention of these infectious diseases by effective immunization programmes.
   You should familiarize yourself with details of common childhood infections by reference to your paediatric textbooks or lecture notes.
   Other vaccinations available for specific individuals and situations include: typhoid, paratyphoid, cholera, yellow-fever, influenza, rabies, and anthrax.
   Vaccination is not normally given to persons who are unwell or in poor health, immunosuppressed, taking steroid medication, undergoing radiotherapy, have reacted to the initial dose, have a significant history of allergic reactions or fitting, or are pregnant.

17.3. Barrier nursing

A patient can be 'barrier nursed' for two main reasons:
1. To protect the patient from the environment.
2. To protect others from the patient.
1. Protecting the patient from the environment is normally referred to as *reverse barrier nursing* and is appropriate for use when patients have a lowered resistance to infection due, for example, to bone marrow

depression, leukaemia, skin loss from extensive burns or when the patient is deliberately immunosuppressed, e.g. following organ transplantation.

2. Protecting others from the patient is used more extensively and there are normally categories of isolation which are defined by the hospital as appropriate to the particular infection. For example,

(a) *strict isolation* involving use of protective clothing and masks would be appropriate for diphtheria;

(b) *respiratory isolation* involving use of masks and correct disposal of tissues and sputum pots would be appropriate for meningococcal meningitis;

(c) *enteric isolation* involving precautions with stools, use of double bagging of linen would be appropriate for salmonella;

(d) *Wound/skin isolation* would be appropriate for wound infections, e.g. gangrene and would involve use of gown, gloves when in contact with the infected wound and correct disposal of any articles such as linen, dressing materials.

Additional precautions may also need to be taken in relation to blood specimens, disposal of needles from patients with suspected serum hepatitis. Key points to consider before barrier nursing a patient are:

1. For what reason is the patient being barrier nursed?
2. Is isolation necessary?
3. Is the degree of isolation appropriate to the infection?

Key aspects of nursing care
1. Preparation of the room/appropriate equipment
2. Explanation to patient, relatives and ward staff about the isolation technique in use
3. Display of appropriate notices
4. Education advice to the patient in relation to hand-washing, cleanliness, general hygiene and specific advice relevant to the particular infection, e.g. importance of covering mouth/nose when coughing or sneezing if the infection is spread by droplets
5. Correct disposal of linen, fomites, urine, faeces, other secretions, and articles which have been in contact with the patient
6. Disinfection and cleaning of the room after the patient is discharged
7. Psychological support relevant to the degree of isolation especially in relation to the patient's fear and anxiety if alone in a side-room.

When answering a question about care of a patient being barrier nursed it is important that you only include appropriate isolation and disposal techniques. Remember that complete isolation is only necessary for highly infectious conditions and then it may only be appropriate for a few days or the initial stages of the patient's illness until antibiotic therapy has taken effect.

Sources of infection include food; H_2O; ventilation systems; dust and dirt; staff and visitors.

Factors associated with susceptibility to infection include nutritional state; age; occupation; illness; medical treatment such as steroids or radiotherapy.

Points to consider when preventing spread of infection are:

1. Do the staff understand the isolation techniques in use?
2. Are there problems with the physical environment?
3. Use of aseptic technique
4. Are the staff carriers? Take appropriate swabs for microscopy, culture and sensitivity.
5. Education about hand-washing, sanitation
6. Involvement of infection control nurse and microbiology department.

17.4. Hepatitis

Key facts
1. Hepatitis is inflammation of the liver.
2. The most important cause is viral infections.

Hepatitis A is transmitted from person to person via a faecal-oral route, e.g. in food or water. The source of the virus can be blood, or saliva. The incubation period is three to five weeks. It is normally a mild infection.

Hepatitis B is transmitted parenterally, e.g. through contaminated syringes or by intimate contact. The source of the virus is blood, saliva or semen. The incubation period is eight to twenty weeks. It is a more severe infection than hepatitis A.

Hepatitis Non-A–Non-B is transmitted via blood transfusion and blood products. The source of the virus is blood. The incubation period is two to sixteen weeks. It can be a very severe infection leading to chronic hepatitis.

Key aspects of nursing management
Patients with ? hepatitis are normally barrier nursed until a diagnosis is confirmed.

Patients with hepatitis A are non-infectious once the jaundice appears and they often do not seek medical help until this stage. Management of these patients is directed at specific problems they present with, e.g., anorexia, lethargy, pruritis. While they are infectious they should be kept on bed rest and special care taken in relation to urine and faeces as these secrete the virus.

Psychological support and explanations as well as creating diversions to relieve the boredom of being on bed rest are important aspects of nursing management. Prior to discharge, advice should be given on hygiene, hand-washing, eating habits as appropriate.

Patients with hepatitis B and hepatitis Non-A–Non-B should remain on bed rest until the hepatitis subsides. They are likely to be more seriously ill and convalescence may take many months. They should be barrier nursed until they are non-infectious and highly infectious carriers must be isolated. Care should be taken with saliva, urine and faeces in case they are contaminated with blood, and specific care must be taken when handling blood specimens.

As with hepatitis A sufferers they will require much psychological support as well as good nutrition and a gradual but progressive mobilization programme back to health.

17.5. Specimen R.G.N. question

Q. Miss Ann Dodds, a 25-year-old travel agency courier, is to be admitted to a medical ward with infective hepatitis. She has a history of anorexia, nausea, vomiting and abdominal pain of several days' duration. Her skin is slightly jaundiced and she is very lethargic.

(*a*) *Outline the measures which must be taken to prevent the spread of this infection.*   25%

(*b*) *Describe in detail the nursing care and management Miss Dodds will require on her admission and during the acute phase of her illness.* 75%

Final R.G.N. paper, English and Welsh National Boards, November 1984

17.6. Multiple choice questions

Q. 1. Which one of the following groups of infections does triple vaccine immunization protect against?

(*a*) *diphtheria, tetanus, poliomyelitis*

(*b*) *diphtheria, whooping cough, poliomyelitis*

(*c*) *poliomyelitis, whooping cough, tetanus*

(*d*) *tetanus, whooping cough, diphtheria.*

The correct answer is (*d*). Protection against poliomyelitis is normally given at the same time but via oral administration of a separate vaccine.

Q. 2. Which one of the following describes the way in which triple vaccine confers immunity?
(*a*) *natural artificial*
(*b*) *passive artificial*
(*c*) *active artificial*
(*d*) *natural passive.*

The correct answer is (*c*). Tetanus and diphtheria vaccines are toxoids and whooping-cough vaccine is made of inactivated organism. They are introduced into the body and stimulate the production of antibodies.

18. Care of patients with visual, hearing and skin problems

18.1. Introduction

Only care relating to commonly encountered visual, hearing and skin
problems is included in this chapter as many students do not have the
opportunity to work in the appropriate specialist units and thus examiners
do not expect a detailed knowledge. If you are training in a hospital which
has a specialist unit caring for patients with eye, ear, nose and throat, or
skin disorders then you should revise these topics in more detail as the
examiners in your hospital would expect you to be more familiar with the
specialist care these patients require.

Management of patients who are deaf and/or blind can be included in
any question as there are many members of the population who suffer
from these problems and are admitted to hospital for treatment of other
unrelated problems. This is especially true of the elderly.

A knowledge of the detailed care of patients suffering from severe burns
or requiring extensive skin grafting or plastic surgery would not be
expected by the examiners but the principles of management of burns and
the initial care and treatment are areas with which you should be familiar.

18.2. Relevant anatomy and physiology

A knowledge of the normal anatomy and physiology of the eye, ear and
skin is necessary in order to understand the principles of care related to
the management of disorders associated with these organs.

The eye

The space in front of the lens is filled with *aqueous humour*.
   The space behind the lens is filled with *vitreous humour*.
   Parasympathetic nerve fibres *constrict* the pupil.
   Sympathetic nerve fibres *dilate* the pupil.
   You should ensure that you revise the function of the eye in relation to focusing as well as consulting your textbook for further details of the parts identified in the diagram (see over).

The ear

You should be able to describe the role of the outer, middle and inner ear in hearing, and the role that the parts identified in the diagram (see over) have in the transmission of sound.
   While revising the above you should also remember to revise the structure and function of the vestibular apparatus in the maintenance of balance.

The skin

The skin is one of the largest organs in the body and its functions are of major importance in the maintenance of homeostasis. In your revision you should include:
1. the structure of the skin: epidermis – the different layers; dermis – the structures located within it
2. colouration of the skin
3. its mechanical properties: tension, compliance, strength
4. its functions: protection, sensation, storage, absorption, heat regulation
5. revision of a diagram of the skin to include:
epidermis
dermis
blood vessels
lymphatic capillaries
sensory nerve endings
sweat glands and their ducts
hair follicles and hairs
sebaceous glands.

The eye (vertical section)

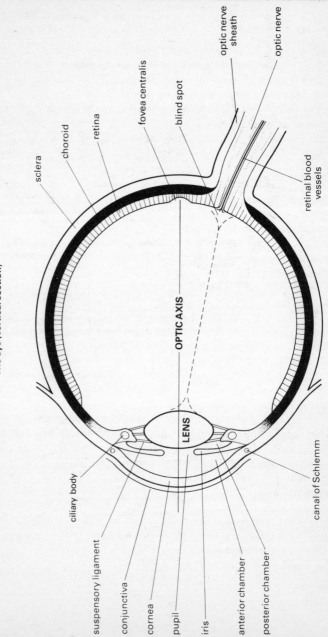

The ear

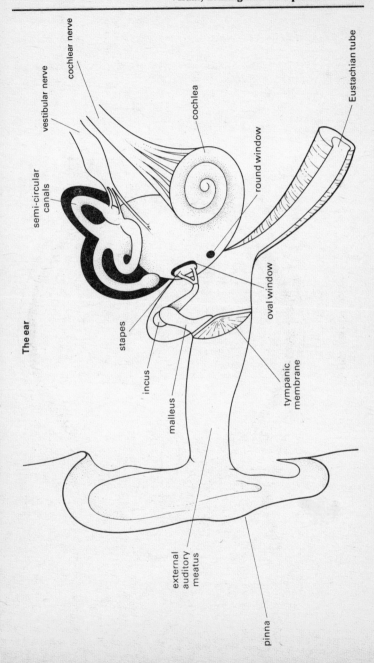

cochlear nerve

vestibular nerve

cochlea

semi-circular canals

round window

Eustachian tube

oval window

stapes

incus

malleus

tympanic membrane

external auditory meatus

pinna

18.3. *Visual problems*

Myopia (short-sightedness) and *hypermetropia* (long-sightedness) are corrected by appropriate spectacles:

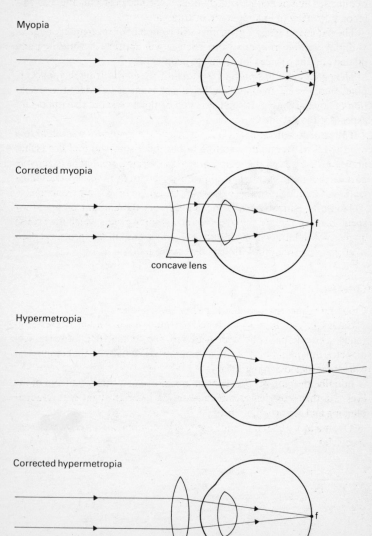

Myopia

Corrected myopia

concave lens

Hypermetropia

Corrected hypermetropia

convex lens

Glaucoma

This is increased intraocular pressure leading to permanent optic nerve damage and blindness. It can be caused by interference with the outflow of aqueous humour either acutely or as a chronic problem, and also as a secondary effect of inflammation or trauma.

The patient with *acute* glaucoma will complain of severe pain, nausea, vomiting and blurring of vision. The eye will appear red with the pupil dilated and the cornea cloudy due to oedema.

The patient requires prompt treatment with *miotic* drugs, e.g. pilocarpine; diuretics, e.g. mannitol and dichlorphenamide to reduce the formation of aqueous humour. Analgesia and complete rest are also important aspects of the patient's care.

The patient with *chronic* glaucoma usually experiences a gradual loss of visual field eventually resulting in blurred vision and dull headaches above the eye and in the temporal region. Surgical treatment to remove part of the iris to facilitate drainage may be used. Long-term administration of miotic drugs is necessary for treatment of chronic glaucoma.

Advice to patients should include limiting the amount of time they spend reading and watching television; avoiding events which may cause an increase in intraocular pressure, e.g. stress, emotional upsets, exertion of energy, constipation with resultant straining.

Cataracts

Clouding of the lens leading to opacity and blindness.

Cataracts can be due to developmental or congenital causes, e.g. following maternal rubella or acquired due to metabolic disease, e.g. diabetes, inflammation or senile degeneration. The latter is the commonest cause of visual loss in the elderly.

Initially, the patient complains of 'mistiness' or a 'speck' in front of his eyes. He then experiences difficulty seeing in bright light with gradual blurring and distortion of vision.

Treatment is the removal of the lens and supplying of compensatory spectacles.

Specific preoperative care
This includes:
1. assessing visual acuity and independence
2. orientation to ward environment
3. psychological preparation for surgery
4. obtaining conjunctival swab for culture
5. administration of prescribed antibiotics to eyes
6. cutting eyelashes
7. administration of mydriatic eyedrops and anaesthetic eyedrops as prescribed prior to operation if local anaesthetic is being used.

Specific postoperative care
This includes:
1. reorientation of patient to surroundings
2. positioning patient on back or unoperated side with bedhead elevated
3. instructing patient to rest and try to avoid coughing or sneezing
4. protecting the eye by use of an eye dressing (shield).

   After the initial period independence should be encouraged. The patient and his family should be involved in instilling the eyedrops if possible. Temporary cataract spectacles may be required and permanent spectacles will be prescribed after approximately six weeks when the eye has settled down.

Blindness

This may result from diseases that interfere with the passage of light, e.g. glaucoma, cataract; impair reception and normal reaction to light, e.g. retinal diseases; interrupt connections with and functions of the cortex, e.g. pressure on the optic nerve, demyelinating and metabolic disorders.

   Points to remember when caring for a blind person in hospital include:
1. Remember he is a normal person who happens to be blind.
2. Do not 'talk down' to him.
3. Introduce yourself when speaking.
4. Address him by name when speaking to him.
5. Orientate him to his locker, bed position and where his possessions are.
6. Tell him what the food on his plate is at mealtimes and where it is located.
7. Do not move items on his locker or leave things for him without telling him they are there.
8. Introduce him to other patients, especially in adjacent beds.

9. Walk slightly in front of him when guiding him and never walk behind him.

10. Do not raise your voice when talking to him unless he is deaf.

11. Encourage independence within the constraints of the ward environment.

Facilities to help blind people include:

Guide Dogs for the Blind

Royal National Institute for the Blind

Department of Health and Social Security – financial benefits

talking books/wireless for the blind

employment services and rehabilitation centres

residential homes, hostels and holiday hotels

provision of braille books, Optacon.

18.4. Hearing problems

Deafness

There are three main causes:

1. External ear obstruction, e.g. the external auditory meatus is obstructed by wax or dirt.

2. Middle ear disease in which the correct functioning of the ossicles is impaired. For example,

nasal catarrh

↓ via Eustachian tube

inflammation of the middle ear (otitis media)

↓

otosclerosis with formation of new bone causing the stapes footplate to become fixed

↓

deafness.

3. Inner ear disease resulting in damage to the cochlear nerve or organ of Corti due for example to trauma, Ménière's disease, infections, e.g. measles, drugs, e.g. gentamicin.

When deafness is due to a failure of the sound waves to be conducted through the outer and middle ear it is known as *conductive* deafness. If the failure is due to damage of the nerve fibres or the cochlea then it is known as *sensori-neural* (or *perceptive*) deafness.

Points to remember when caring for a deaf person in hospital include:

1. Assess the degree of deafness so as to plan care appropriately.

2. Always face the deaf person so he can see your face clearly.

3. Do not cover your mouth with your hand.

4. Speak slowly and clearly.

5. When talking or listening to the patient pay full attention and do not become distracted.

6. Ensure that he has understood what you are saying.

7. If necessary, write down messages to him.

8. Always check to ensure his hearing aid (if used) is working correctly and the batteries are charged.

9. Do not shout or raise your voice unnecessarily.

10. Take into account the feelings of isolation, loneliness, insecurity and suspicion that the person may have especially if he is elderly and in a strange environment.

11. Try to understand his speech but if this is not possible ask him to write messages to you.

12. Never pretend you have understood him when you have not.

Facilities to help the deaf include:

Royal National Institute for the Deaf

Department of Health and Social Security – welfare benefits

special education for children

'hard of hearing' clubs

modifications to television, telephone, doorbell

help to learn to lipread, use hand signs

hearing aids for conductive deafness.

18.5. Skin problems

If you have worked in specialist dermatological units then you should refer to your lecture notes for details of specific conditions and their nursing management. The points below are those which a nurse on a general ward should consider if a person with a skin disorder such as eczema or psoriasis is admitted for treatment of a different problem.

1. Greet the patient in a normal way, e.g. shake his hand.

2. Do *not* express revulsion or distaste.

3. Remember how anxious the person will be about his appearance and having to be admitted to hospital.

4. Ensure appropriate privacy is provided.

5. Discuss with the patient any treatment he is having for the disorder and facilitate his being able to continue this, e.g. application of specific ointments.

6. Discourage him from scratching lesions.

7. Familiarize yourself with details of the specific disorder he has so as to plan the most effective nursing management.

8. Do not isolate him or treat him differently from other patients.

9. Administer any prescribed treatment and if this includes steroid therapy observe specifically for side effects of this.

10. Promote good hygiene and diet.

18.6. Burns

Key facts

Burns are classified by:

1. *Depth*:

(a) Superficial (first degree) involving destruction of the epidermis

(b) Partial thickness (second degree) involving destruction of the epidermis and part of the dermis

(c) Full thickness (third degree) involving destruction of the epidermis, dermis and sometimes subcutaneous tissue, muscle and bone.

2. *Area*: for example, using Wallace's Rule of Nines.

See p. 290.

Principles of first aid management

1. Removing the cause of the burn

2. Placing person in a comfortable position

3. Protecting burnt areas

4. Summoning medical help and arranging transfer of person to hospital

5. Placing burns in cold water to prevent further tissue damage should only be used if the burn is less than 9 per cent.

Physiological problems associated with acute burns

These include:

1. fluid loss through wound into the extracellular space as oedema

2. fluid loss beneath the surface as blister fluid

3. fluid loss via the wound to the surface as exudate.

Reduction of the circulating blood volume as a result of the above may lead to shock. The remaining circulating fluid becomes concentrated with red blood cells – haemoconcentration.

Shock results in: decreased metabolism; decreased body temperature; reduced renal function; muscular weakness.

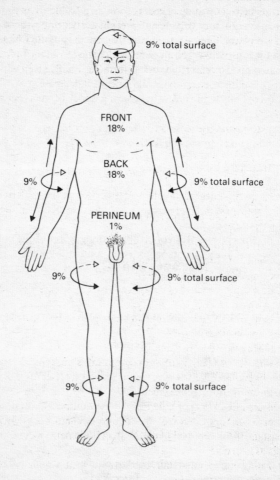

9% total surface

FRONT
18%

BACK
18%

9%

9% total surface

PERINEUM
1%

9%

9% total surface

9%

9% total surface

Principles of treatment in a 'shock case'
1. Resuscitation (as appropriate)
2. Fluid replacement commenced as soon as possible so as to maintain an adequate circulatory volume and prevent the development of shock.

Fluid is replaced by oral and intravenous route at a rate which is never less than the rate of loss. The amount is calculated from the time of injury and is based on a special replacement formula. Fluids given will contain a balance of colloids, electrolytes and 5 per cent dextrose.
3. Control of body temperature by ensuring 'shock room' is between, e.g. 26°C and 29.5°C
4. Anticipation and prevention of respiratory problems
5. Prevention and control of infection
6. Relief of pain and anxiety.

Points 1 to 4 are vital in order to prevent irreversible shock and death occurring.

Key aspects of nursing management
These should include:
1. Preparation of room and equipment for receiving patient
2. Availability of barrier nursing equipment
3. Recording of vital signs, height, weight
4. Assessment for evidence of complications, e.g. respiratory failure
5. Strict asepsis
6. Obtaining history to enable nursing-care plan to be constructed
7. Checking for other injuries
8. Administering prescribed analgesia
9. Assisting with setting up of intravenous infusion, central venous line, intravenous cut-down procedure, volumetric control pumps, e.g. Tekmar, to ensure accurate fluid replacement
10. Accurate monitoring of fluid intake, urine output, haematocrit
11. Observation for evidence of overloading circulation or dehydration
12. Assistance with removal of clothing, debridement, wound toilet and dressings as instructed
13. Informing patient and relatives of nursing action being taken including appropriate explanations.

After initial care the patient would normally be transferred to a burns unit (unless suffering from a minor burn) for further treatment and skin grafting. If you have nursed patients in these areas in your hospital then you should refer to your notes and relate these to your experience so that you are prepared for answering a question – if asked – about nursing care of a burnt patient during the exposure, surgical and rehabilitation phases.

18.7. Specimen R.G.N. question

Q. Mrs Elsie Cobb, aged 50 years, is brought by ambulance to the accident and emergency department having sustained burns to her trunk and upper limbs in a gas explosion at her home.

(a) Describe the nurse's role in the reception and initial care of Mrs Cobb.
60%

(b) Explain why fluid replacement is important while Mrs Cobb is in the accident and emergency department and outline the related nursing care she will be given.
40%

Final R.G.N. Paper, English and Welsh National Boards, January 1985

19. Care of the dying patient

19.1. Introduction

When you are asked to discuss care of a dying person, this will usually refer to someone in the last stages of malignant disease although occasionally the patient will be suffering from another condition such as renal failure. It is important that you are aware of the specific problems that different kinds of cancer produce according to the organs affected, e.g. nutritional difficulties caused by oesophageal or gastric malignancy.

In most cases you will be concerned not only with the *total* care of the patient but also that of his family as the two cannot be separated.

An example of a recent R.G.N. question is:

Q.2. Mr George Allen, a 52-year-old father of three children, has a long history of renal disease. He is admitted with uraemia and is unconscious and very dehydrated.

Using a problem-solving approach, discuss the care which would be appropriate for Mr Allen and his family during the last few days of his life.
100%

Final R.G.N. paper, English and Welsh National Board, July 1984

Another guiding principle to bear in mind is that although you should identify all the patient's needs and problems, the care goals you set are not related to recovery or an improvement in his condition but towards maintaining his physical, emotional and spiritual comfort and enabling him to come to a peaceful and painfree death.

19.2. Attitudes

Death is still very much a taboo subject and most people feel embarrassed and afraid of open discussion about it. There are many occasions when a dying person would like to ask questions or talk about his impending death but is inhibited from doing so by the knowledge that this would not be considered acceptable. Research has shown that nursing staff tend to have less interaction with dying patients in hospital than with other patients who are likely to recover.

Relatives are often concerned that the patient should not be told the truth about his condition because they feel that he could not cope with it; patients often insist that relatives are not told for the same reason. It is not normally the nurse's responsibility to decide who should be told and how much, but it is very important that she knows to what extent the patient and his family are aware of his dying state and she should avoid encouraging a conspiracy of silence unless *all* carers are convinced that this really is in the best interests of the patient. Too often it is the carers who cannot cope with the reality and therefore cannot allow the patient the opportunity to do so.

The reaction of a person to the news that he is dying is completely individual and you must never assume that advanced age, prolonged suffering or unhappy social circumstances make approaching death more welcome to some people than others.

A fairly consistent pattern of responses to the knowledge that a person is terminally ill has been identified mainly through the work of Elizabeth Kubler-Ross. She identified a pattern of:

denial or disbelief

anger

bargaining

depression

acceptance.

These responses are shown in varying degrees not only by the dying person but by all those (including professionals) who are involved in his care. You must remember, however, that not everyone who is involved will go through these stages at the same rate and, unhappily, not all of them will reach the stage of acceptance.

It is very important that the nurse recognizes what stage the individual has reached in his emotional responses and makes her care appropriate to the needs engendered by that particular state of mind.

19.3. Needs

The patient

As long as the patient is alive he has the same full range of needs that every other person has. With reference to Maslow's hierarchy of needs (see Chapter 5, pp. 80–81), the dying person still needs to have the basic physiological and emotional needs satisfied before he can be helped to the ultimate self-actualization of understanding and accepting his impending death, but particular emphasis should be placed on the need for love and the need for self-esteem. The loneliness of the dying person is one of the most difficult problems to overcome.

In addition to meeting the needs explicitly related to his dying condition you must ensure that the patient is:

1. free from pain and discomfort (whether or not this is associated with his terminal illness)
2. adequately nourished and has enough to drink
3. clean and fresh and presenting a body image acceptable to him
4. able to eliminate without discomfort or humiliation
5. involved as much as possible in decisions affecting his care
6. in an environment which provides variety and distractions to the extent that he wishes it
7. provided with relaxed and considerate company and communication
8. given the opportunity to fulfil his spiritual requirements.

The patient's family

'Family' must include not only immediate blood relations but those people (and sometimes animals) to whom the patient relates and feels closest.

The family, too, in this stressful situation still have the full requirement of needs. In many cases, the predominating need expressed is the need to be able to *do* something.

1. Encourage, allow and assist family members to share in the care as much as they wish.
2. Make sure that when they do help they are shown how to do things and where things are.
3. Provide privacy for the patient and his family to be together.
4. Ensure that rest and refreshment facilities are made available.
5. Give family members time and opportunity to talk through their own feelings and ask questions.
6. Make sure that appropriate help and accurate information is given

with regard to financial difficulties, social problems and the practicalities involved when someone dies.

7. Provide comfort and support until and when the patient dies but also ensure that provision is made for family support as necessary after the bereavement.

Nurses and professional carers

1. The death of the patient must not be seen as a failure; a positive attitude towards care of a dying person must be cultivated and encouraged.

2. The nurses themselves may grieve and must be allowed to share their grief among themselves and with the patient's family.

3. There is often a need to discuss and evaluate the care given after the death of a patient.

4. The carers must trust and support one another.

19.4. Pain and symptom control

Pain control is often considered to be the key to all care of a dying person. The patient must not only be free from pain but free from the fear of pain.

The first consideration is an adequate analgesic régime. This is the responsibility of the doctor, but the nurse must monitor and provide information as to its effectiveness. Analgesia – which can almost always be taken orally – must be given absolutely regularly and on time. Medication must not be withheld because the patient is not yet experiencing a recurrence of pain. It is important to provide a régime which gives the patient freedom from pain without clouding of consciousness.

The effectiveness of pain relief is greatly enhanced if the patient is handled gently, positioned comfortably and is neither too hot nor too cold. If alcoholic drinks assist in promoting a feeling of wellbeing, they should be encouraged in moderate quantities.

Much of a dying person's distress is often caused by failure to deal with other uncomfortable problems. The nurse must ensure that the patient does not suffer from any of the following:

dry and dirty mouth
dirty eyes
soreness from incontinence
constipation
pressure sores
hunger/thirst.

Simple medical measures can alleviate the problems caused by nausea, coughing and respiratory distress, or unpleasant smells from discharging wounds or orifices.

The patient's mental state will interact with his bodily comfort and if he is feeling loved, able to express his hopes and fears, and at peace with himself, the physical care given will be made more effective.

19.5. Where to care

There are three main options to consider when deciding where a dying person should be cared for: home, hospital, or hospice.

Home

Advantages:
Familiar surroundings and belongings
Continuity of family life
Privacy
Maintenance of independence.
Disadvantages:
Stress on family carers and disruption of home life
No one at home to care
Possible lack of adequate physical facilities, e.g. cramped surroundings
Skilled nursing care not always available.

Ideally, it is best for someone to be able to spend his last days loved and cared for at home but for this to be possible it is essential that adequate back-up services and facilities are provided and that community care team members work together with the family to achieve this end.

Hospital

Advantages:
Twenty-four-hour skilled nursing and medical care
Full nursing and medical resources available
Reduced family burden.
Disadvantages:
Loss of privacy and independence
It may be difficult for family to visit
The patient is made constantly aware of his condition.

Hospice

Advantages:
Specialist skill constantly available
Relaxed, comfortable environment
Admission is often on a 'relief from home' or 'symptom control' basis.
There is usually very good home back-up and communication.
Disadvantages:
Limited number of places available – sometimes a waiting list
It may be a long way from home
It is exclusively devoted to the care of dying people.

19.6. Care of the terminally ill child

This is an emotionally stressful time for all – parents, child, staff and other children in the ward. The following are general points to remember.
1. You are nursing the whole family, not just the dying child.
2. Allow the parents to do as much as possible for the child, so that they do not feel they have failed.
3. Spend time with the parents to build up a relationship, so that they can ask questions and express their feelings.
4. Keep some normality in the daily routine so the child is not too bewildered by what is happening to him.
5. Try to understand the emotions of the parents who will be working through the stages of bereavement.
6. Recognize expressions of anger and hostility towards the staff for what they really are, and accept them without retaliation.
7. Understand the emotions of the child who knows of his prognosis and will also be experiencing the emotional responses to dying.
8. Be aware of the concept of death held by the child, depending on his age and past experiences.
9. Answer the child's questions simply and directly, in an appropriate way for his age and level of thinking.
10. Listen to the child, and allow him to express his feelings and fantasies in play, stories or art.
11. Respond to the questions of other children honestly and appropriately; assure them (where this is the case) that the same thing will not happen to them.

To achieve all of this it is necessary for the nurse to come to terms with her own attitudes and feelings about death. When caring for terminally ill children, nurses also need the support of each other.

19.7. Sample question and answer

Q. Mrs Louise Finlay, a 56-year-old married lady, has been cared for at home by her husband and their daughter who lives with them. Mrs Finlay has an advanced lung cancer and is very dyspnoeic and emaciated. She and the family are aware of the diagnosis.

Using a problem-solving approach describe the nursing care and management Mrs Finlay will require following her admission to hospital for terminal care until her death. 100%

Mrs Finlay will obviously need a high level of nursing care and attention and it is important in an answer to this type of question to allocate an appropriate amount of your answer to the care required in relation to the most significant problems, e.g. dyspnoea, cough, pain, anxiety, fear.

1. *Dyspnoea*: Well-ventilated position in the ward, not draughty but near to window. Sitting upright to facilitate easier breathing, either in a chair or in bed and well supported with pillows. Administration of prescribed, humidified oxygen and appropriate drugs to relieve bronchospasm, e.g. salbutamol via nebulizer. Reduce respiratory demands by ensuring that things Mrs Finlay needs are near to her bedside and she thus does not need to take unnecessary physical activity.

2. *Cough/sputum*: Provide sputum pot, tissues and bag within easy reach and change regularly. Administer prescribed expectorants in order to help facilitate the removal of secretions or promote sleep as appropriate. Arrange gentle chest physiotherapy to help with breathing and expectorating. If she smokes, try to discourage her but not if this will increase her stress/anxiety levels. Oropharyngeal suction may be necessary to remove secretions in the later stages of her care.

3. *Pain*: Ensure adequate analgesia is prescribed and administer it regularly to maintain constant circulating drug levels in the blood. Ensure patient is as comfortable as possible as this will enhance the effect of the analgesia.

4. *Anxiety/fear*: Be available to listen and talk to Mrs Finlay and her family about their fears and anxieties. Remember, they may be experiencing the bereavement process at different rates and take this into account when talking to them. Make appropriate referrals for counselling/support to, for example, specialist cancer counsellors. Provide spiritual support if required. Encourage her family and friends to be with Mrs Finlay whenever they wish. Ensure that comfort and support is provided at night as this is often the time that most patients feel frightened and alone.

5. *Awareness of approaching death*: It is important to allow a patient to say goodbye by encouraging communication and affection with the family. Do not leave Mrs Finlay alone and ensure that privacy is maintained for her and her family. If the presence of a priest will help her to die in peace then facilitate this.

The above represent the most important problems to include in your answer. However in a 100 per cent answer of this type you would also be expected to outline care in relation to the other physical problems which Mrs Finlay would be experiencing. For example:

1. *Difficulty in taking adequate food and fluids*: Provision of small, frequent, nourishing drinks of choice and small amounts of food when she desires it.

2. *Loss of independence in personal hygiene*: Providing help as needed for regular bed bath and washes as well as ensuring that hair, nails and dentures are not neglected. Involve Mrs Finlay's daughter and her husband if they wish.

3. *Dry mouth*: Providing frequent mouthwashes and latterly oral toilet so as to reduce the risk of fungal infection, promote comfort and offset the drying effect of oxygen.

4. *Reduced mobility*: Ensure frequent changes of position, use pressure-relieving devices, e.g. sheepskin; handle gently and provide gentle physiotherapy in order to promote comfort and reduce the risk of pressure sores.

20. The examination

The night before

Try to relax and have a good night's sleep. You will have done the necessary study and revision by now and may only confuse yourself by trying to cram more information in at the last minute. Also, you need your energy for the next day.

Examination day

1. Get up in good time to ensure you can get to the examination centre without having to rush.
2. Try and have something to eat for breakfast.
3. Take something, e.g. sweets or glucose tablets, to suck during the examination in case you are hungry.
4. Make sure you take your entry card with you.
5. Take pens, pencils, ruler and a rubber with you.
6. Try to use the toilet before entering the examination room.
7. Follow the registration/admission procedure for the examination as directed at the centre.

In the examination room

1. Arrange your pens, etc, in front of you on your desk and leave your other belongings at the place directed by the invigilator.
2. Settle yourself as comfortably as you can at your desk.
3. Place your entry card on the desk so the invigilator can check it during the examination.
4. Listen to the invigilator's instructions and follow them carefully.
5. Read and comply with the instructions on the front cover of the examination book. This will vary depending on the type of examination. For example, for multiple choice questions,

(a) Fill in your candidate number.

(b) Use only the pencil provided.

(c) Do not use a rubber.

(d) Alter answers only in accordance with the instructions.

It is usually best to answer all the questions to which you believe you know the correct answer and then to return to those you are less sure of. Try not to guess but to eliminate the distractors logically.

For the essay paper:

(a) Make sure you know how many questions you have to answer.

(b) Divide your time equally allowing for planning your answers.

(c) Read ALL the questions on the examination paper.

(d) Choose your questions and decide on your order of answering.

(e) Plan your answers taking into account the guidelines in Chapter 1.

(f) Start a fresh question at the appropriate time. Do not spend longer on your first answers. You can always return and add more if you have time left at the end.

(g) Start a fresh question on a fresh page.

(h) Do not be deterred or distracted by what other candidates are doing. Concentrate on your own answers. Remember, you will only gain marks for information the examiners asked for and not for irrelevant or additional material, even if it is correct.

Good luck!

FOR THE BEST IN PAPERBACKS, LOOK FOR THE 🐧

PENGUIN PASSNOTES

This comprehensive series, designed to help O-level, GCSE and CSE students, includes:

SUBJECTS
Biology
Chemistry
Economics
English Language
Geography
Human Biology
Mathematics
Modern Mathematics
Modern World History
Narrative Poems
Nursing
Physics

SHAKESPEARE
As You Like It
Henry IV, Part I
Henry V
Julius Caesar
Macbeth
The Merchant of Venice
A Midsummer Night's Dream
Romeo and Juliet
Twelfth Night

LITERATURE
Arms and the Man
Cider With Rosie
Great Expectations
Jane Eyre
Kes
Lord of the Flies
A Man for All Seasons
The Mayor of Casterbridge
My Family and Other Animals
Pride and Prejudice
The Prologue to The Canterbury
    Tales
Pygmalion
Saint Joan
She Stoops to Conquer
Silas Marner
To Kill a Mockingbird
War of the Worlds
The Woman in White
Wuthering Heights

FOR THE BEST IN PAPERBACKS, LOOK FOR THE

In every corner of the world, on every subject under the sun, Penguin represents quality and variety – the very best in publishing today.

For complete information about books available from Penguin – including Pelicans, Puffins, Peregrines and Penguin Classics – and how to order them, write to us at the appropriate address below. Please note that for copyright reasons the selection of books varies from country to country.

In the United Kingdom: For a complete list of books available from Penguin in the U.K., please write to *Dept E.P., Penguin Books Ltd, Harmondsworth, Middlesex, UB7 0DA*

In the United States: For a complete list of books available from Penguin in the U.S., please write to *Dept BA, Penguin, 299 Murray Hill Parkway, East Rutherford, New Jersey 07073*

In Canada: For a complete list of books available from Penguin in Canada, please write to *Penguin Books Canada Ltd, 2801 John Street, Markham, Ontario L3R 1B4*

In Australia: For a complete list of books available from Penguin in Australia, please write to the *Marketing Department, Penguin Books Australia Ltd, P.O. Box 257, Ringwood, Victoria 3134*

In New Zealand: For a complete list of books available from Penguin in New Zealand, please write to the *Marketing Department, Penguin Books (NZ) Ltd, Private Bag, Takapuna, Auckland 9*

In India: For a complete list of books available from Penguin, please write to *Penguin Overseas Ltd, 706 Eros Apartments, 56 Nehru Place, New Delhi, 110019*

In Holland: For a complete list of books available from Penguin in Holland, please write to *Penguin Books Nederland B.V., Postbus 195, NL–1380AD Weesp, Netherlands*

In Germany: For a complete list of books available from Penguin, please write to *Penguin Books Ltd, Friedrichstrasse 10 – 12, D–6000 Frankfurt Main 1, Federal Republic of Germany*

In Spain: For a complete list of books available from Penguin in Spain, please write to *Longman Penguin España, Calle San Nicolas 15, E–28013 Madrid, Spain*